Cancer Saved My Life

Cancer Saved My Life

Lois Berry

Writers Club Press
San Jose New York Lincoln Shanghai

Cancer Saved My Life

Writers Club Press
an imprint of iUniverse.com, Inc.

For information address:
iUniverse.com, Inc.
5220 S 16th, Ste. 200
Lincoln, NE 68512
www.iuniverse.com

ISBN: 0-595-14969-3

Printed in the United States of America

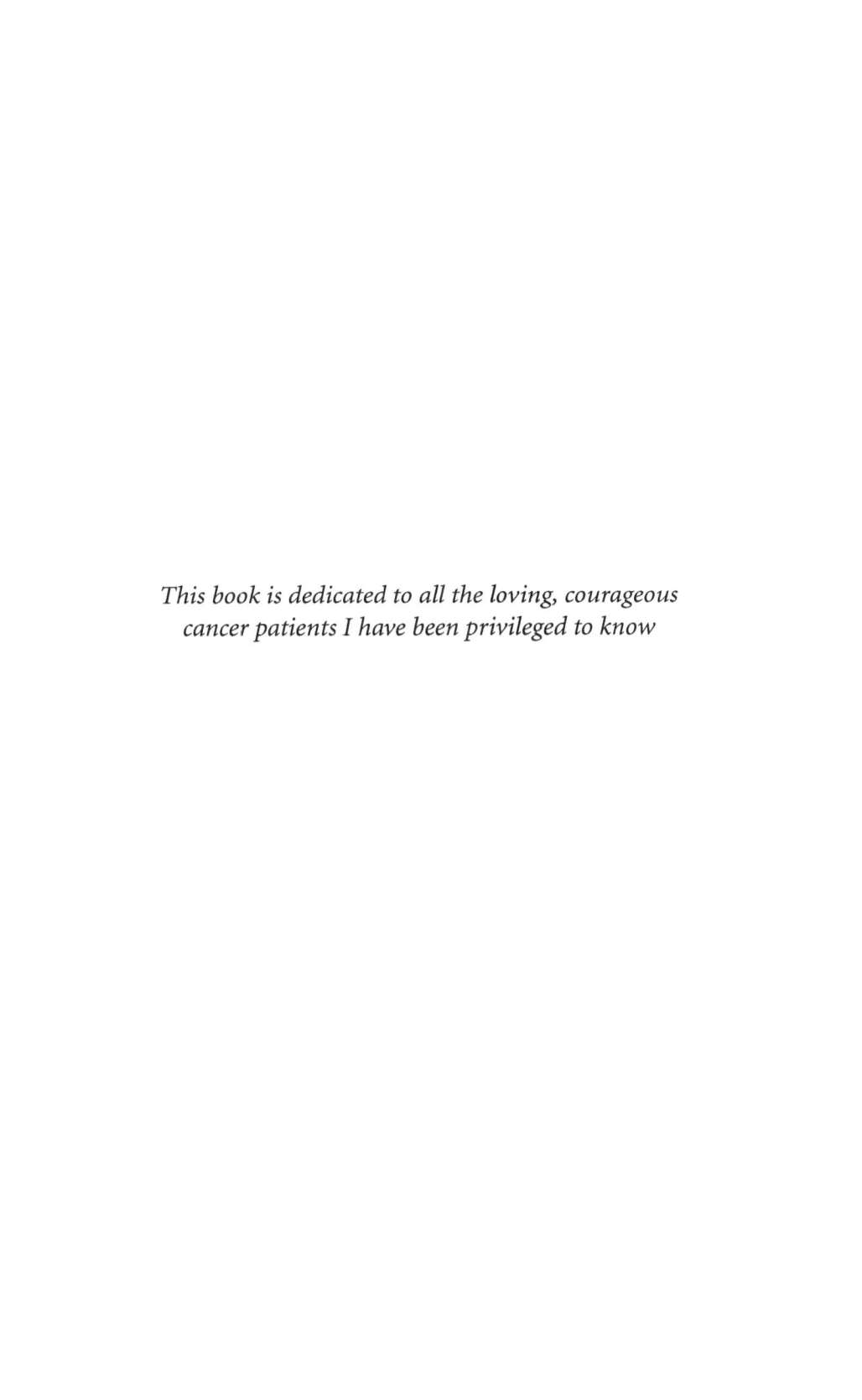

*This book is dedicated to all the loving, courageous
cancer patients I have been privileged to know*

Contents

Acknowledgements

I am deeply indebted to the following people:

To my sister and editor, Ruth Bennett. She has been my confidant and faithful friend for a lifetime.

To my daughter, Jody Meredith, for her helpful suggestions and contribution.

To my daughter-in-law, Chris Berry, for her contribution to this book.

To daughter, Ruth Cogswell, for her contribution and to her husband, Chris, and my son, Jim for their unfailing support.

To my daughter, Barb Berry, who insisted that I learn to use a computer and for the hours of lessons it took to make me computer competent. Without her help, I would not have been able to write this book.

To my grandson, Jeff, who helped me put my presentation together.

To John Bennett for his contribution.

To Dr. Glenn Warner, my oncologist and friend. His love and devotion to his patients is unparalleled. His medical expertise was responsible for my surviving cancer. His belief in treating not only the disease but also the whole person changed my life and started me on the road to wellness.

To my other grandchildren, Kelly, Jaime, Ronee, Mark and, Jenn for believing in me.

Finally, to all the wonderful people who have made my life such a joy.

Introduction

Anyone who has heard a doctor say, "You have cancer," knows the fear that fills your heart and mind. I was no exception and originally I certainly didn't consider it a blessing. It was a long time before I realized it had changed my life for the better.

When I was diagnosed with breast cancer in 1969, I thought it was a a death sentence. People spoke in hushed tones around me. I had no knowledge of the disease or treatment. Such a diagnosis turned my world upside down.

After a radical mastectomy, it was four years later when my cancer had metastasized to the bone and I was in dire trouble, that the real fight to survive began. Since that time, I have learned so much and come to believe that having cancer resulted in my making changes that have contributed to a happier, healthier long life. From my vantage point today, I look on cancer as a gift. I began this journey in ignorance. The word "cancer" was not even in my vocabulary. Along the way, I learned that my participation was essential if I was going to survive. It was not enough to present myself to a doctor and say, "Cure me," without making changes in my lifestyle which included both mind and body.

I would like to share with you what I've learned in the hope that it will assist you in your recovery. Your experience may be different, but however we get there we cannot live the rest of our lives being afraid every day. During the course of this book, I will discuss reading material that I found helpful. It is always good to read about others who have recovered from this frightening disease and learn from their experience. There are many good books written about positive thinking. They tell us that there is a proven relationship between how we think and how we feel. They tell us to be positive instead of being negative, to be happy, to learn to handle stress, to eliminate fear, but they don't always tell us how to accomplish these things. It isn't easy but it is worth the effort to work toward goals that eventually bring us to a happy, productive life.

I am going to tell you exactly how I arrived at this stage of my life as a very longtime survivor of cancer and hope it will help you on your journey to wellness in both body and spirit. I don't pretend to be an expert, but I have learned a great deal over the years and would like to pass it along to you in the hope that it will help you to be healthier and happier.

One of the most important things I have learned is that we are all in this journey through life together. We need to be there for one another with love and compassion.

So, this is my story.

Chapter I

That Dreaded Diagnosis—Cancer

I was experiencing an intermittent pain in my right breast so I made an appointment to see a gynecologist. The doctor I had been going to for years and who had delivered three of my four children had retired. The new doctor came highly recommended and this would be my first visit. When he examined my right breast, he said he found a lump. In a very gruff voice he asked me how long this had been going on. When I replied that I had experienced the pain for a week or ten days he said, "Well, you have cancer and that breast will have to come off."

This doctor didn't know me, had no idea how I would react to such news, and apparently didn't care. I was stunned and in a state of shock as I left his office. Suffice it to say, that was my one and only visit to his office.

In the years since, I have often wondered what made this doctor act toward me in such a brutal manner. Until I went for an examination, I was healthy except for a slightly annoying pain in my breast. I think it would have been possible for him to have eased me into what lay ahead for me in a much more gentle way. He could have said that there seemed to be something suspicious and that I should see a surgeon about the possibility of a biopsy.

After I came home from the doctor's office, I called a surgeon who was also a good friend. It was a Friday and he could not see me until Monday, but told me to keep busy and try not to think about it, excellent advice but impossible to follow after such devastating news. The mind simply does not work that way. Mine kept repeating, "You have cancer, you have cancer, you have cancer."

I spent a little time trying to get my emotions under control. Then I told my husband and children what had transpired. I don't recall that any of them said a word. It seems they just sat there in stunned silence. I thought I was doing OK—my husband and I even played bridge with the neighbors as I thought it would keep my mind off my difficulties. During the night, I woke up sick to my stomach and started vomiting. I was so ill the rest of the weekend I couldn't eat. This had nothing to do with my cancer, but rather the fear that consumed me.

On Monday, I had my appointment with the surgeon and his calm manner reassured me. He told me he was 98% sure the lump was only a benign tumor and that he would schedule a biopsy on Wednesday to confirm his opinion. In contrast to my examination with the first doctor, this consultation did wonders for my mental attitude. I went home feeling good again and ate a big lunch. This was example number one of the effect the mind has over the body. In the years since, there has been much written about the mind/body connection, but at that time the medical community gave no credence to the power of the mind in maintaining a healthy body.

Thirty years ago the patient with breast cancer had no options. I was required to sign a release form before going to surgery stating that if the biopsy showed a malignancy, I agreed to a radical mastectomy. This is debilitating surgery that not only removes the breast but chest muscle and all the lymph nodes under the arm. In the years since, it has been proven by numerous studies that a lumpectomy (removal of the tumor) or a partial mastectomy (removal of the lump and part of the breast) are equally effective. A sampling of the lymph nodes instead of the removal of all of them is sufficient to detect if the cancer has spread from the breast. In fact, in reports I later received from the Congressional Subcommittee on Health it was apparent that the continued use of radical mastectomies had been in question for over twenty-five years. It was the first example I had of how very slow the medical profession is to change.

I remember waking up in my hospital room and seeing my husband and sister standing by my bed. It's amazing how vividly certain events remain in our memory. I recall thinking that they wouldn't tell me if I had cancer. Instead, I asked them what time it was. I knew what time I had gone to surgery for the biopsy and somehow my brain was telling me that if I had been in surgery for several hours, I had cancer. I determined that was true and drifted back to sleep. I awoke to the surgeon shaking me awake. I looked at him and said, "How about that lousy 2%!" The surgeon told me at that time that he sent samples to be biopsied twice because he had been so sure that the tumor was benign.

I had my first example of positive thinking in relation to cancer as I lay in my hospital bed. I made a mental list of all the things I would hate to lose and discovered that one breast came way down the list. For instance, the loss of my eyesight, hearing, arms or legs would be far more devastating. Implants were not a common procedure in those days and I never really considered it as an option. I had a prosthesis made but it was so big and bulky that I never wore it. In fact, it was bigger than the remaining breast and made me look lopsided. Finally, I gave it away.

After recovering from the radical surgery, I simply went on with my life as before. The surgeon said, "I got it all." Now I know that he should have said, "I got all I could see." The lymph nodes showed no spread of the cancer and I was not referred to an oncologist. No treatment was recommended, but it was suggested that I have regular checkups with an internist.

The internist I selected later became head of oncology at a local hospital and that is a scary thought as he did not show any particular skills taking care of me. In fact, during our visits he talked more about his own difficulties practicing medicine then he did about any problems I might have. His examinations were not very thorough and he always pronounced me in good health. He made no suggestions about lifestyle such as diet, exercise or mental attitude. After I had been seeing him for several years, he wrote me a letter saying I was cured. In retrospect, this letter was amazing because I had been telling him for some time about a pain I was experiencing in the pelvic area which apparently he never heard because he was not listening to me.

Even with my background of breast cancer, this doctor didn't even bother to take an x-ray. As the pain persisted, I made an appointment to see my surgeon. As soon as I told him about the pain, he ordered x-rays of the area. I waited while the film was developed and it showed a growth on or in the bone.

One of the problems I encountered at this stage of my ongoing struggle with cancer was not only my own fear, but also the fear of those around me. It was so real that I could feel it from family and friends even though they didn't voice their concerns.

At the time, I remember a great sadness. My oldest daughter who lived in Washington, D.C. was pregnant with her first child. It would be my first grandchild. I realized that there was a good possibility that I would never see my grandchildren grow up. My daughter was so upset by my latest diagnosis that we had to fly her home so she could see me and talk to my doctor. Not only did I live to see that grandchild, but I have five more. I feel so privileged to have been involved in their lives and watch them grow up.

After my day of prayer which I explain in the chapter titled *Spiritual Renewal*, my fear was completely gone, but I could still feel it in those around me. At this time, I asked my husband and four children to get up in the morning and think of me as well because that was what I was doing every day. I was claiming a complete healing. Also, I tried to distance myself from others who were negative. It is extremely important to surround yourself with positive people

I went into the hospital for a biopsy which showed that the breast cancer had metastasized to the bone. Because the surgeon believed my cancer was estrogen produced, they also did tests to see if my ovaries were producing estrogen and would have surgically removed them if this had been true. It was also at this time that I was referred to the doctor who changed my life.

I remember so clearly being wheeled from my hospital room downstairs to the Tumor Institute of Swedish Hospital in Seattle, WA. I sat in an examining room for quite awhile, but finally I had my first encounter with Dr. Glenn Warner. It is hard to explain what this man brought to his practice of medicine. He was intelligent and knowledgeable. But more than that he had such a loving and calming manner and was able to communicate that he really cared. He didn't minimize the seriousness of my cancer, but said that working together we could overcome the problem. He gave me HOPE as he did with all patients. He expected a great deal from his patients and I will discuss that later.

During that first visit, he said he would like to treat me with immunotherapy. I didn't have a clue as to what that entailed. However, his explanation sounded good to me. Immunotherapy attempts to build up the body rather than tearing it down with toxic chemotherapy drugs. My medical treatment consisted of the use of Bacillus Calumette Guerin (BCG) and a male hormone, Teslac.

BCG is a vaccine used for many years as a treatment for tuberculosis. It is still considered experimental for all cancers except bladder. In correspondence I have had with the Food & Drug Administration (FDA), they informed me that BCG has not been released from the Investigative New Drug (IND) list because no pharmaceutical company has ever requested its removal. When I inquired why that was, they told me it was because it was an inexpensive product and the drug companies couldn't make money selling it. It is still available and is what the FDA calls an "off shelf" drug which means it is approved for certain usage, but it is perfectly legal for other applications at the physicians discretion. It is usually administered by scratching a grid on the skin, applying the BCG and covering with a patch for 24 hours. Much like any vaccination, the patient usually runs a low grade temperature for 24 hours. It was the only side effect I ever had. I don't recall how many of these treatments I received, but they were given over a period of months: first, every week, then every two weeks and so on, extending the time intervals until the course of treatment was completed.

During the course of the treatment, I was never ill and was able to lead a perfectly normal life. I had periodic bone scans for several years and my cancer never spread any further then the one area on the pelvic bone. I believe that if I had been given conventional therapy (radiation and/or chemotherapy) I would not have survived.

At that particular time when I knew so little about cancer treatments, I could have been easily persuaded to use any treatment my doctor suggested. In those days, I thought doctors were all knowing. I do not think that way anymore. Doctors are well meaning but they certainly don't know all the answers. Patients should do their own research and ask questions and if they are not satisfied with the response they receive, they should find a doctor whose recommended treatment and philosophy are compatible with their own beliefs.

When I think back, it is frightening to think how trusting I was at that time. Now I truly believe that God was watching out for me and directed my surgeon to send me to the one doctor who saved my life.

Months after I started treatment, I ran into my internist at a store. I thought he would be so pleased to know that I was doing well, especially after missing the diagnosis of my breast cancer metastasizing to the bone. The first surprise was that he obviously did not even know who I was so I had to refresh his memory. Then when I told him how well I was doing on immunotherapy treatment expecting he would be pleased, he spent the next fifteen minutes telling me I was making a terrible mistake. I couldn't believe it. It is possible that he could have learned something about less invasive and debilitating ways to treat cancer, but he had an absolutely closed mind.

When we get over the initial shock of being a cancer patient, we need to marshal all of our resources and the help of others to overcome our fears. Fear weakens our immune system and impedes the healing process.

What I learned through this experience has affected all areas of my life. It has made me more compassionate of others. It has taught me that what is really important are my relationships with family and friends; loving and being loved.

Chapter II

Immunotherapy

For those readers who are not familiar with the differences between so-called conventional therapy and immunotherapy, a discussion of the treatment and philosophy may be helpful at this point. Radiation and chemotherapy kill both sick cells and healthy cells in an attempt to eradicate the cancer. Immunotherapy uses natural substances in an effort to stimulate the immune system to fight the cancer. Both disciplines will usually recommend surgery to remove as much of the tumor mass as possible which gives the body's defense mechanisms a better opportunity to deal with the cancer that is left after surgery. Treating the whole person with changes in lifestyle along with medical intervention is an important part of the immunotherapy approach.

Surgery, radiation and chemotherapy have been the standard treatment for cancer for many years. Yet, even 100 years ago there were medical oncologists and scientific researchers who were investigating the mysteries of the body's own immune mechanisms. Most diseases, including cancer, are the result of the immune system malfunctioning. So what exactly is known about the immune system? Through years of study and discoveries by many different research scientists, the structure of the immune system is pretty much understood. What seems to elude the sci-entific world is how to duplicate the efforts of our body's immune responses to repair such deficiencies as occur in cancer.

We do know that if we did not have an immune system we would die of the slightest infection. Each of us has a network of cells and organs that work together to defend the body against attacks by foreign invaders. These are primarily germs—tiny infection causing organisms such as bacteria and viruses, as well as parasites and fungi. Germs or microbes try to break into the human body because it provides an ideal environment. It is the immune systems job to keep them out or, failing that, to seek them out and destroy them. When the immune system mis-fires, however, or when it is crippled, it can unleash a torrent of diseases.

The immune system is amazingly complex. It can recognize millions of different enemies, and it can produce secretions and cells to match up with and wipe out each one of them. The secret to its success is an elaborate and dynamic communications network: millions and mil-lions of cells, organized into sets and subsets, pass information back and forth like clouds of bees swarming around a hive. Once immune cells receive the alarm, they undergo strategic changes and begin to produce powerful chemicals. These substances allow the cells to regulate their own growth and behavior, enlist their fellows, and direct new recruits to trouble spots. At the heart of the immune system is a remarkable ability to distinguish between the body's own cells (self) and foreign cells (nonself). The body's immune defenses normally coexist peacefully with cells that carry distinctive "self" marker molecules. But when immune defenders encounter cells or organisms carrying markers that say "foreign", they quickly swing into action.

Immune cells and foreign particles enter the lymph nodes via incom-ing lymphatic vessels or the lymph nodes' tiny blood vessels. Once in the bloodstream, they are transported to tissues throughout the body. They patrol everywhere looking for foreign antigens, then gradually drift back into the lymphatic system, to begin the cycle all over again.

The immune system stockpiles a huge arsenal of cells, not only lymphocytes but also cell-devouring phagocytes and their relatives. Some immune cells communicate by direct physical contact, sometimes by releasing chemical messengers.

In order to have room for all the cells needed to match millions of possible enemies, the immune system stores just a few of each kind. These few matching cells multiply into a full-scale army when needed. After their job is done, they fade away.

How does the body mount an immune response? Microbes attempting to get into the body must first move past the body's external armor. The skin and the membranes lining the body's gateways not only pose a physical barrier, they are also rich in scavenger cells and IgA (Immunoglobulin G) antibodies. Next, invaders must escape a series of *nonspecific* defenses that are normally ready to attack.

Microbes that cross the nonspecific barriers must then confront *specific* weapons tailored just for them. Specific weapons, which include antibodies and cells, are equipped with singular receptor structures that allow them to recognize and interact with their designated targets.

Long ago, physicians realized that people who had recovered from the plague would never get it again—they had acquired immunity. This is because whenever T cells and B cells are activated, some of the cells become *memory cells*. The next time that an individual meets up with the same antigen, the immune system is set to demolish it.

Immunity can be strong or weak, short-lived or long-lasting, depending on the type of antigen, the amount of antigen, and the route by which it enters the body. Immunity can also be influenced by the genes you inherit. When faced with the same antigen, some individuals will respond forcefully, others, feebly, and some, not at all.

An immune response can be sparked not only by infection but also by immunization with vaccines. *Vaccines* contain microorganisms—or parts of microorganisms—that have been treated so they will be able to provoke an immune response but not full-blown disease.

The cells of the immune system, like other cells, can grow uncontrollably and the result is cancer. *Leukemias* are caused by the proliferation of white blood cells, or leukocytes. The uncontrolled growth of antibody-producing plasma cells can lead to *multiple myeloma*. Cancers of the lymphoid organs, known as *lymphomas*, include Hodgkins disease.

The immune system provides one of the body's main defenses against cancer. When normal cells turn into cancer cells, some of the antigens on their surface may change. These new or altered antigens can flag immune defenders, including killer T cells, natural killer cells, and macrophages. According to one theory, patrolling cells of the immune system provide body wide surveillance, spying out and eliminating cells that become cancerous. Tumors develop when the system breaks down or is overwhelmed.

Evidence is mounting that the immune system and the nervous system are linked in several ways. One well known connection involves the adrenal glands. In response to stress messages from the brain, the adrenal glands release hormones into the blood. In addition to helping a person respond to emergencies by mobilizing the body's energy reserves, these "stress hormones" can stifle the effects of antibodies and lymphocytes.

Hormones and other chemicals known to convey messages among nerve cells have been found to "speak" to cells of the immune system. Indeed, some immune cells are able to manufacture typical nerve cell products, while some lymphokines can transmit information to the nervous system. In addition, the brain may send messages to the immune system directly, down nerve cells. Also, networks of nerve fibers have been found connecting to the lymphoid organs.

Because of the possibility that you are not familiar with words used in the above discussion of the immune system, the following are brief explanations.

The organs of the immune system are positioned throughout the body. They are called *lymphoid organs* because they are home to the *lymphocytes* that are small white blood cells, key players in the immune system. The lymphocytes travel throughout the body, using either the blood vessels or their own lymphatic vessels. They are the main types of immune cells and B and T cells are the main types of lymphocytes. *B cells* work chiefly by secreting soluble substances called *antibodies* into the body's fluids. Antibodies ambush antigens circulating in the bloodstream, but are powerless to penetrate cells. I think it is interesting that each B cell is programmed to make one specific antibody. For example, one B cell will make an antibody that blocks a virus that causes the common cold, while another produces an antibody that attacks the bacterium that causes pneumonia and so on.

The job of attacking target cells—either cells that have been infected by viruses or cells that have been distorted by cancer—is left to the *T lymphocytes* or other immune cells. They work primarily by secreting potent chemical messages known as *cytokines* or, more specifically, *lymphokines*. Binding to target cells, lymphokines mobilize many other cells and substances. They encourage the growth of cells, trigger cell activity, direct cell traffic, and arouse phagocytes.

Phagocytes are large white cells that can swallow and digest microbes and other foreign particles. *Monocytes* are phagocytes that circulate in the blood. When monocytes migrate into tissues, they develop into macrophages. Specialized types of macrophages can be found in many organs, including the lungs, kidneys, brain, and liver.

Natural killer cells (NK cells) are another kind of lethal white cell, or lymphocyte. Like killer T cells, NK cells are armed with granules filled with potent chemicals. However, killer T cells attack only their specific matching targets, natural killer cells attack any foe. Both kinds of killer cells slay on contact. The deadly assassin binds to its target, aims its weapons, and then delivers a lethal burst of chemicals.

Substances known as biological response modifiers can be used to bolster the patient's immune response. These include BCG (Bacillus Calmette Guerin) and, more recently, interferon and interleukins. Interferon and interleukins are manufactured in the body, but are not there in sufficient quantities when the immune system is weak. They can be given to bolster the body's defense system or to enhance any other treatment given to the patient. As I mentioned in discussing my treatment with BCG, it has been approved for the treatment of tuberculosis for many years. It is applied like a vaccine on the surface of the skin (scarification) or injected directly into the body.

After all these years of demonstrated benefits, BCG is still considered experimental for all cancers except bladder. The approval for the use of BCG in the treatment of bladder cancer came about because 1,600 urologists petitioned the FDA requesting that it be removed from their IND (Investigative New Drug) list. It is what is called an off-shelf drug and is available to doctors to use as they deem appropriate. However, because it is still on the FDA IND list, insurance companies will not pay if it is used as a treatment in most cancers. In conversations with the FDA, they told me that they believed that BCG is a harmless drug and had no problem with its use. It saddens me to think of how many patients might have benefited from this safe, inexpensive, non-toxic drug.

For more information on immunotherapy or where this treatment might be available, you can log on to the Internet. The National Institutes of Health can be found at http:/www.nih.gov/

The National Institutes of Health also has a toll free number—1-800-422-6237

Chapter III

Getting Started on the Road to Recovery

Perhaps the most important decision to be made is the selection of our doctor. This is a life and death matter and it is essential that our oncologist is a person who believes that our recovery depends on a partnership of mutual respect and understanding, a doctor who believes that you, the patient, needs to take charge of your recovery. We need the doctor for his medical expertise, but he cannot do it alone as there are many changes we can make to facilitate our wellness.

I remember a young girl who was diagnosed with ovarian cancer. She set up appointments with seven oncologists and she interviewed each one. All but one recommended the same treatment—chemotherapy. The seventh suggested a less invasive approach with the lifestyle changes that are so important to getting well and staying well.

She asked each doctor to give her the names of five ovarian cancer patients who had survived their recommended treatment for at least five years. Only the seventh doctor was willing to do so. The others cited patient confidentiality which makes me laugh and it makes me wonder whether they had any patients that had survived for at least five years. I have talked to hundreds of cancer patients and their family members over the years and am always happy to do so. Anyone I know who has survived cancer is eager to share the good news.

It didn't take long for my young friend to pick the one oncologist who offered her something other than toxic drugs. I saw her often for many months and she never suffered any side effects while she was being treated. Even more important, she is alive and well many years later. (Under standard treatment, the cure rate for ovarian cancer is low).

I have learned that *once a cancer patient, always a cancer patient.* By this I mean that as cancer patients we must always be vigilant about our health. When we are first diagnosed, we will do anything to get well. Later, when we seem to be free of disease, we slack off, and that is when we get into trouble again. Our health should become a lifetime commitment.

I find that people are much more knowledgeable about cancer today and are searching for the kind of care that will allow them still to have a life. They have heard such horror stories about the debilitating effects of the treatment that they are often more fearful of that than they are of the disease.

As I have said, when I began this odyssey as a cancer patient, I was totally ignorant of the disease. I was one of those people who pretty much thought that the doctor knew what was best for me and didn't question anything. I would have done anything the surgeon told me to do after my breast cancer metastasized to the bone. He was the one who referred me to the doctor who took a totally different approach to my cancer and I know it saved my life. I believe it was another miracle.

Now let us assume that you have selected an oncologist who will work with you and listen to your concerns. It is possible that you will need surgery to remove the tumor mass. Removing as much of the tumor as the surgeon can see will give your immune system a better chance to eliminate any remaining cancer cells. (This is true except in the case of prostate cancer where the removal of the encapsulated tumor often spreads cancer cells to other parts of the body). This risk, in addition to the troubling side effects, is not worth taking.

Experts tell us that everyone has cancer cells in his body, but most of the time our marvelously complex and efficient immune system keeps them under control. When our immune system is suppressed, it becomes overwhelmed and that is when we get into trouble.

It makes sense then to do everything we can to boost the capabilities of our immune system. This will not only keep us free of cancer, but will lead to a much healthier life. Since I have had cancer, I am in better health than I ever was previous to that time. So how do we accomplish this.

Chapter IV

Steps to a Healthier Life

VITAMINS

I have been on a program of megadoses of vitamins and supplements for years. These were prescribed by my doctor and are reviewed periodically. I am going to list them for you to give you some idea of what such a program includes. *I am not suggesting that this is exactly what you will need.* Consult with your doctor or a naturopath to decide what is right for you.

Some of the supplements are obvious for my particular need. For instance, because my breast cancer was estrogen produced and metastasized to the bone, I take large amounts of calcium and magnesium.

Vitamin C—(Ascorbic Acid Crystals)—4,000 milligrams per day. 2,000 milligrams in morning and 2,000 evening.

Vitamin E—1600 IU per day. 800 IU in the morning and 800 IU evening.

Oyster Shell Calcium—1500 mg. 500 milligrams morning, noon and night.

A *Therapeutic Formula* containing vitamins A, C, D, E, B6, B12, Thiamin, Riboflavin, Niacin, Folate, biotin, Pantothenic Acid, Zinc, Selenium, Manganese and Chromium. There are small amounts of each drug in this formula so in addition I take larger quantities of the following:

Beta Carotene—60 mg. Per day. One 30 mg. tablet in the morning and another at night.

Selenium—25 mg. One per day.

Co-Enzyme Q10—10 mg. One per day

Zinc Picolinate—30 mg. One per day.

Chromium Picolinate—100 mg. One per day.

Magnesium Complex—150 mg. One per day

Aspirin—1/2 per day.

DIET

My doctor was advocating changes in diet for his patients long before it was accepted by anyone in the medical profession. Even today, many physicians believe it has nothing to do with wellness. How could that be? Surely, what we put into our bodies will affect our health. It just seems like common sense.

There is some agreement today that a low fat, essentially sugar free diet is beneficial not only for cancer patients but heart patients as well. Some people adopt what is called a vegan diet. They do not eat any meat (including chicken and fish) or any dairy products. Their diets consist of pastas, rice, vegetables, fruits, grains and soy products.

There are many variations of diets most of which I think are so restrictive that it would be very difficult to remain on them for any length of time. I believe that as we are making changes we can do it gradually and not make radical changes that we find impossible to stick with for the long term. We need to be comfortable with the choices we make.

I gradually became a vegetarian and I find that easy to maintain. After years of cooking for a family and serving red meat more often than chicken or fish, I find that I don't miss red meat at all. I think your taste buds must change over time. Now, if I had to eat a hamburger, I think I would choke. I do eat chicken and fish but only about twice a week. Most of the time, my diet consists of rice, pasta or potatoes, vegetables, fruit and grains such as oatmeal and whole wheat bread. I like soups and there are many already prepared that are available at the grocery store and are meat free; i.e. minestrone and vegetarian vegetable. I use almost no milk and very little cheese products. I use a powdered, tasteless soy product for additional protein which I add to my morning oatmeal. I'll admit to a sweet tooth and I do eat some sugar. Perhaps what I eat will help you in deciding a healthy diet.

I have never used juicing in addition to other dietary changes. However, many cancer patients I know are convinced that this practice has contributed to their recovery. It certainly can't hurt to try it. If you would like to start on such a program, either talk to someone who does juice or go to the library for information

As a reference, I have used "New Choices in Natural Healing", edited by Bill Gottlieb and published by Prevention magazine. This book cites the guidelines of Cherie Calbom, M.S., a certified nutritionist in Kirkland, Washington and the co-author of "Juicing for Life".

Calbom emphasizes that choosing a juicer is the first important step. She says the best values are in the $100 to $200 price range and should have 0.4 horsepower. She prefers a machine that ejects the pulp out one side and pours the juice from the other. Above all, she states, the juicer should be easy to clean. If it's a hassle to clean, you will tend not to use it. She also prefers a machine that breaks down into four dishwasher safe parts.

EXERCISE

Why is it so hard to stick to a program of exercise? I know it is for me, but I know it is essential to keep my body fine tuned. This is especially true as we get older whether or not we have or have had cancer. We need to fit an exercise program to our capabilities and our limitations, if any. It certainly is not going to do any good to set up an overly ambitious program for yourself if you're in a constant state of anxiety because your goals are too high. Start slowly and build on your successes. The main thing is to keep moving. A sedentary life is not good for any of us.

There are many forms of exercise that are beneficial; walking, running, swimming, aerobics, gardening, dancing and bicycling, to name a few. If you do better in organized group activities, then sign up to participate several times a week. For some, exercising with others encourages you to keep going and the camaraderie is helpful. Or, do it on your own. I walk and do stairs. One of the benefits of walking is that it doesn't cost anything.

I often have the following conversation with myself. "I'm too busy today, too much to do, I don't have time." And then I say to myself, "Stop making excuses. It only takes 1/2 hour and I waste more time in a day than that." So get going—you'll feel so much better and it will give you a boost mentally.

These are steps we can take to improve our physical well being. If you feel good physically, you will feel better emotionally. Our emotional well being is every bit as important as our physical health. In fact, in my opinion, it is difficult to separate one from the other.

Chapter V

Relaxation Techniques

BIOFEEDBACK is based on the assumption that it is possible to exert a certain amount of conscious control over bodily functions ruled by the nervous system. These functions are identified as heart rate, skin temperature and respiration. Instruments are attached to the body that make visual or audible any variations in these physiological activities so the patient can see or hear what is going on in his own body. Patients have learned to reduce high blood pressure, eliminate migraine headaches, control irregular heartbeats, increase and decrease blood flow. It would seem to me that this technique would require complete concentration by the patient and the ability to visualize what is occurring in the body.

HYPNOSIS is really just a state of focused concentration. Whether clinically or self-induced, it produces an altered state of mind. A patient in a state of hypnosis is amenable to suggestion. I have always been skeptical of the benefits of hypnosis, but as I have read more on the subject I wonder if we don't all practice self-hypnosis.

How do we react to bad news? Do we have a positive or negative mental approach to life? Do we think the best or the worst of people and events? Are we optimistic and enthusiastic about life? Or, on the other hand, are we always expecting the worst to happen and when it does do we say, "Why me?"

I know the mind has a powerful effect on the body and if we can turn negative attitudes into positive ones, it will affect our health. How do we do that?

It seems that some people are just born with an optimistic nature, but it can be cultivated. I remember listening to an interview with Beverly Sills, the internationally known opera singer. I had always admired her bubbly personality. Ms Sills had experienced many tragedies in her life and the interviewer said to her, "How do you manage to always be so happy?" She replied, "I'm not always happy but I choose to be cheerful." Some people go through life as victims. Others refuse to be defeated by life and circumstances.

I believe that we can change our attitudes by constant attention to what we are thinking and perhaps that is self-hypnosis.

MEDITATION and self-hypnosis seem to be closely associated. Meditation is described as a going within yourself or learning to be completely quiet. With practice, it is possible to clear your mind and retreat to a place of peacefulness. Prayer would seem to me to be a form of meditation. What you are trying to find is stillness. Everyone has a different experience, but what you are attempting to accomplish is an ability to relax your mind.

YOGA is similar to meditation, as it can heighten your awareness of your physical, mental and emotional state. It is the state of harmony and the means of realizing it, which links the individual to the universal self. How yoga differs from meditation is the physical aspect. The yoga instructor will first take you through deep breathing exercises and relaxation techniques. There are dozens of poses that are designed to stretch and strengthen the muscles, improve posture and the skeletal system, massage internal organs and stimulate the nerves. There are different recommended poses for particular health problems that have evolved over centuries of their use. Your instructor should be aware of your physical limitations and not allow you to push your body beyond its capacity. Medical research has shown that many techniques are potent, therapeutic instruments. They can restore health to an ailing body, to some extent slow the aging process, and even reverse some of its effects.

ACUPUNCTURE is performed by a specialist in this method by placing needles into the body at key points. The patient usually feels no pain and there are no side effects. As most of you probably know, Chinese doctors and their patients have been using this method of healing for many centuries. They believe the body is a series of energy conduits called Chi. This energy flows along systemic meridians that do not coincide with any known physiologic structures. The acupuncturist is looking for hidden forces that are out of balance. In the last decade or so, this method has gained wider acceptance in Western medicine.

ACUPRESSURE works on the same principle as acupuncture, but uses the hands instead of needles.

TAI CHI is also an ancient Chinese art and looks like a dance as the participants gently and effortlessly sway weaving their arms, legs, torsos, feet, hands and heads in gentle motion. The Chinese do not call it a dance or exercise. It is about harmony and tapping into a source called chi.

Other relaxation techniques include *massage, aromatherapy*, the use of a system of caring for the body with botanical oils, and *reflexology*, a way to healing through manipulation of the feet.

It is certainly possible to change the way you think and feel without participating in any of the above, but any technique that works for you is good. Change is a gradual thing. Remember that you are trying to change habits of a lifetime so be patient with yourself. You may need to try several disciplines before you find what is most comfortable for you. What each of us is striving for in any relaxation techniques, is an inner peace.

When I first had cancer thirty years ago, there wasn't much offered other then medical intervention. There was little recognition of the connection between the mind and the body. Today there are many books on the subject. When I first started on my road to recovery, I had to search for books that had any positive outlook for cancer patients. The ones I did read were a tremendous help to me in changing my attitudes.

If you decide to try any of the structured techniques to help you relax, be sure to give it ample time to work. I have seen patients jump from one thing to another with no benefit from anything. When we are first diagnosed with cancer, we are so fearful and so anxious that it's hard to make decisions about care. Everyone is telling us what to do and we end up even more confused and anxious.

We need to take the time to work out a program that fits our capabilities and needs. What works for one person does not necessarily work for another. You may want to try several different approaches before you decide what is best for you. Above all, you *must believe in what you are doing to get well.*

When we first have cancer, selecting a doctor, deciding on a treatment program and using these other techniques are the first essential steps. We need to feel comfortable with and believe in the choices we make.

Medical intervention is important and I do not want to minimize that in any way. However, I do believe that we will never be completely well unless we can honestly evaluate and correct the emotional problems in our lives.

Chapter VI

Spiritual Renewal

My treatment didn't stop with the medical intervention. Dr. Warner believed that just treating the disease was not enough, that it was imperative to treat the whole person and to do this the patient's participation was essential. There have been many books and articles written in the last few years that support this concept. However, in 1973 this was a very novel idea and certainly not supported by the medical community. In fact, even today the majority of doctors resist the involvement with their patients that is necessary to assist them in getting well in both body and mind.

Before the diagnosis of bone cancer was confirmed, I spent a day alone and in prayer. I realized later that I did not pray for the cancer to be taken away, but rather for the strength and dignity to meet whatever lay ahead for me. I didn't want to fall apart as I had when I was told I had breast cancer. On that day, God said to me, "I am here; I have always been here" and I realized that He never deserts us, we desert Him. This presence is always available to us, but we need to ask for it.

I remember that on that day I finally surrendered my ego to God. I had experienced numerous crisis situations in my life and was proud of the fact that "I" was always able to cope. There was a lot of "I" did this and "I" did that in my life. No more. In this life threatening situation, I finally said, "I cannot do this anymore by myself and I turn my life and my ego over to you, God."

The next day was amazing. I felt as if a light was flooding around me all day and I had an inner peace that I had never known before. All fear of my cancer was completely gone. Since that time, I have come to believe that each of us is an instrument of God and, if we will let Him, He works through us to accomplish good. None of us ever uses all of our potential and talents, but if we will listen to that Higher Power it will direct us to accomplish things we never thought possible. We need to ask for direction and then we need to *listen*. This applies not only to our health but to all aspects of our life. We are all so busy that we don't have any quiet time and we certainly are not going to be given direction unless we clear our minds of all other distractions. God will work through us in every area of our life if we will let Him.

Just a small example to explain what I now believe. My small church needed to build a new parsonage. The project dragged along until I was nudged to take charge. Some of the members thought I was overstepping my authority and I guess they were right. However, my inner voice kept telling me it was possible and at little or no cost to the congregation.

Somehow, I received permission from the minister and trustees to start this project. There certainly was much skepticism amongst the congregation. We could sell the present parsonage which I felt would cover most of the cost. The first miracle was that a member of the church stepped forward and paid off the small existing mortgage on this property.

Naysayers told me that you couldn't build a house by committee. I selected three people to work with me and we hired a contractor we didn't know. His wife was a member of our church and that seemed recommendation enough to me. We needed a bridge loan and at the suggestion of one of the committee members, we asked if church members would be interested in loaning us the money with a small interest rate for six months. It was over subscribed in two weeks.

A beautiful house was completed in four months on property the church owned and we never had an argument about any aspect of the construction. If we had a disagreement, we voted and the majority ruled. In fact, we had such a good time we were all sorry when the parsonage was finished. I wrote the contractor a thank you note because he was responsible for every aspect of this building and even donated much of his time and talent. He told me it was the first thank you note he had ever received for a building project and I replied, "Well, maybe it's the first time you have been involved in a project where God was in charge."

Up until the time I turned my life completely over to God, my religious life had been sort of off and on. I attended the Christian Science church as a youngster and as a young adult. After some devastating events in my life, I turned from religion entirely. It wasn't until sometime after my marriage that I began to go to church again. I certainly thought I was a Christian and I use that word advisedly because there are many people of other faiths who believe in a Supreme Being. I liked being in church because it was a peaceful, loving place to be, but there was always something missing. I felt an inner void, a longing for something more. I had so many unanswered questions that no one seemed able to answer to my satisfaction. At that time, I read many books on the subject of religion and had philosophical discussions with people of faith.

I spent a great deal of time with a wonderful retired minister and he helped me along on my quest. One day I said to him, "I wish I had your faith." And he replied, "Keep working on it because it takes a lifetime." It wasn't until my day in prayer after my diagnosis of bone cancer that the light finally dawned. I did not need the answers to all of my philosophical questions. I only needed trust. On that day, I was freely given faith by the grace of God. It was certainly not anything I had earned. It has been an awesome presence in my life ever since. That was the first gift I received because I had cancer and there have been many others. Today I can truly say that cancer blessed my life.

One of the most important lessons in my spiritual development has been learning to release the past so that I can live fully in the now. I know that I bring my past with me to any new beginning, but I choose to take only whatever adds to my enrichment and growth. I carry with me the understanding I have gained from my experiences, but I let go of the excess baggage of guilt and regret.

As I do this, I gain greater knowledge from each new experience. God is continually giving me new understanding and the opportunity for a new beginning. I release myself and others from limitations and mistakes of the past. I *choose* to let go of yesterday's mistakes and begin anew.

Chapter VII

Forgiveness—Self and Others

Hatred is a physically damaging emotion. Every one of us needs to forgive in order to be a whole person. If we examine our innermost feelings honestly, each of us will find past hurts, times when we feel we were treated unfairly, hatred of ourselves or others. How do we deal with these feelings?

The deepest need all of us undoubtedly have is the need to forgive ourselves. For what you may say?.

1. Do you ever think about things you've said or done that you wish you had handled differently?

2. Have you ever spoken in anger and wished you could take back the words that came out of your mouth?

3. Do you dwell on past mistakes until they make you miserable?

4. Have you ever criticized unfairly or been judgmental without knowing the facts?

5. Have you ever been engaged in such destructive behavior that you can't get over the guilt and the shame?

6. Are you unable to forgive real or imagined slights?

If we examine our past, I think all of us will find things we regret. Maybe we have not even realized that we have been allowing these regrets to foster and damage our self-esteem. Those of us who have raised children can always look back and see things we wished we had handled with more wisdom. I tell myself that I did the best I could with the wisdom I had at the time.

Certainly, we cannot change the past so it is absolutely non-productive to keep beating ourselves up over past actions we regret. We need to learn from any mistakes and go forward resolving to do a better job in the future. We need to start loving those in our lives with a love that is unconditional. *And we need to start loving ourselves!*

What is unconditional love? It is easy to love those who are always loving to us. What is more difficult in relationships is to keep on loving family or friends who disappoint us. My sister said to me once, "Why is it that the child that is the most unlovable is the one who needs the most love?" It is of the utmost importance that the person who disappoints us knows that we are not going to withdraw our love. In other words, I will only love you if you are good. We do not have to condone the behavior, but we can forgive it.

One of the ways to control our anger and keep ourselves from saying hurtful things to others is to take a time out. When both parties have had time to cool off, set a time to sit down and discuss your differences. It has always made me laugh when I read articles that tell us to argue intelligently. Who does that? The trouble with arguing is that most of us do not stick to the subject of contention. In our anger, we dredge up all kinds of past slights and hurts. We say things that the other person will always remember and find difficult to forgive and forget.

Loving and commitments are hard work sometimes. Of course, we can refuse to risk any close relationships in order to avoid the possibility of being hurt, but that would result in a very empty life. It takes a lot of love and courage to make commitments. It takes loving and forgiving to stay the course in good times and bad times. It is impossible to hold ourselves blameless in all situations. Even so, we need to love ourselves and others with all of our imperfections.

I know people who go through life as victims. They will recite every bad thing that has happened to them given any opportunity. Everything conspires against them and they are miserable. They are convinced that the world is against them and never take responsibility for their own actions. They can always find someone to blame for their mistakes and bad choices. They will tell you that nobody likes them and that may be true because they aren't much fun to be around.

On the other hand, I know people who have survived and prospered against incredible odds and are living their lives with hope and joy. They are loving and forgiving people. Their life experiences have not made them bitter. On the contrary, they have learned so much and are empathetic with the problems of others.

I recently read a remarkable story of forgiveness in the Seattle Times (July 21, 2000) by staff reporter Eli Sanders. It is a too familiar story of four teenagers drinking and driving too fast. The police said the car, driven by Kalani Plunkett, was going 110 miles per hour before it crashed killing one of the passengers, Danny Asrari. The parents are grieving the loss of their child. They say they have become fearful and overly protective of their other children.

What is remarkable to me is the ability of this family to forgive. The father of Danny said that an attorney had told them they should file a civil suit against the family of the driver. He rejected that idea because he does not see much meaning in the prevailing notion that monetary compensation heals all wounds. He feels that the guilt the parents of the driver must feel is enough.

The mother of the driver is quoted as saying, "It's awful. I think about Asraris. I can't even speak. I am just a bundle of nerves. I just feel for them. Their son is dead and my son is alive. Words cannot express the sorrow I feel for them."

As Plunkett awaits his sentencing on vehicular homicide, the parents of Danny believe the judge needs to be firm. Then the mother adds this statement, "Kalani, he needs to be thankful that he's alive. For him to heal, he needs to serve the jail time. Let him pay his dues, and then I hope he has a good life. I hope his parents have a good life."

In reading this account of forgiveness, I wonder how I would react in a similar situation. In tragedies like this, normal reactions besides grief are bitterness and anger. To be able to overcome these negative emotions, is a major step toward healing.

Forgiving others for real or imagined hurts is actually self-serving. Being angry with another probably is not hurting that other person at all. Often, they are not even aware of what they did to hurt us or do not care. However, being angry is hurting me both emotionally and physically. I can feel the change in my body when I start thinking about some long ago hurtful episode in my life. If I continue to dwell on it, it can make me sad and physically ill.

There are events in our lives over which we have no control that change the course of our existence. Then, there are many things and events over which we do have control and the choices we make determine how we live. We can even choose to be happy. I, for one, am determined to live my life with as much joy as possible. I am not perfect and my life isn't perfect, but I would rather count my blessings than dwell on the negatives. I am so grateful that my family and friends accept and love me in spite of my imperfections. I try to do the same in return.

I don't know the author, but there's a little saying I like to repeat each morning as I start the day. It goes like this, "Be accepting of relationships as they are. Know that each person in my life is doing the best they can. Know that I can change me—not them."

I would also like to recommend the book "Forgive and Forget" by Lewis B. Smedes. It is the best I have read on this subject. Refer to the chapter on recommended reading for more information on this book.

Chapter VIII

Dealing with Stress

All of the things we have discussed such as choosing your doctor, diet, exercise, positive attitude and spiritual renewal are important. However, we have to deal positively with the stress in our lives if we are to gain total health physically and emotionally. In fact, I believe that learning how to resolve stressful situations in my life is the most important lesson I have learned. *It is absolutely essential to our mental and physical health.*

Over the years, I had always believed that I handled problems well. I found out that I was wrong. In examining past stressful situations, I didn't always resolve them; I stuffed them. In situations that needed to be addressed, I too often kept quiet because I disliked confrontation. I let real or imagined wrongs fester inside of me. I thought of myself as a peacekeeper and that took a toll on my physical and emotional well being. I came to realize that I was tense a good deal of the time.

I have learned that we have to come to terms with our emotions somehow. There are ways, especially within a family, to allow yourself and others to express their anger and frustration without it becoming a shouting match. Call a time out if the discussion becomes too heated.

However, it is OK to let others know when their behavior is unacceptable to you. It is important that those involved know that you love them, but you are disappointed in their actions.

We need to realize that we cannot eliminate stress. It's how we react to stress that is the difference. I have a friend who said to me, "Life without stress is stressful." He is a high powered, Type A personality who is a problem solver and wants to be in control. I am not that type of person. I want serenity and inner peace in my life and I have worked hard to achieve that goal.

Where do we begin? Initially, I believe we must make an honest evaluation of our lives. From an early age, I had experienced tragedies and difficulties and realized that I had never resolved many of them. I always took great pride in the fact that "I" could cope and go on with my life.

As an example, my mother was killed in an automobile accident when I was thirteen years old. Her death left two very young girls to take care of an invalid father and an ailing grandmother. I remember being so angry at my mother for dying and I certainly could not understand a God who would let that happen. In those days, no counseling was available to help us sort out our feelings and we could not have afforded it if there had been. The subject of my mother's death was never discussed at home. Each person in the family simply nurtured his own grief and I was confused, angry and fearful for a very long time.

We were expected to go on with living the best we could and in some ways that was OK, but, on the other hand, it was years before I came to terms with that terrible tragedy in our lives.

Years later I was able to talk through the hurt and anger with a minister friend and he convinced me that God is not responsible for accidents. I do now believe that a loving God grieves with us. I still do not understand why it happened and never will, but I do accept.

There is always a great sadness that I didn't have a Mother growing up and that she never knew her grandchildren. It took a long time, but I now accept the fact that many things are beyond our understanding.

In our relationships, if a particular person is making us unhappy with his behavior we have to do one of three things: talk to him, release him or eliminate him from our lives. The last suggestion sounds drastic and is not always possible. However, whenever feasible I surround myself with positive, loving people.

I have good self esteem. I like myself and think I'm an OK person most of the time. Because of this, when someone is angry or raises their voice to me, I think *they* have a problem. My immediate reaction is, "Why are they mad at me? I haven't done anything that deserves being yelled at." The majority of the time I'm right. I just happen to be an easy target for the person that is angry and yelling.

I love the story of the husband who has had a bad day at the office. He comes in the door and yells at his wife, she in turn yells at her daughter who yells at her brother who then yells at his little sister and she kicks the cat. Who has the problem here? I would say it was the husband who couldn't confront the situation at the office.

We are all searching for inner peace and joy in our lives. We travel different paths in achieving serenity. Mine came on that day when I was diagnosed with bone cancer and finally turned my life and ego over to God. I cannot imagine living without the belief that there is a Higher Power that is guiding me and protecting me. I am not self-sufficient; I am constantly asking for guidance and I thank God for every good thing in my life.

I know that religion is often a touchy subject, but I urge you to find a church and attend regularly. Even before I was given faith by the grace of God, I found church to be a peaceful, soothing place to be quiet. I consider my church to be a part of my support system. The people there are wonderful and loving and have become a big part of my life. I know I could call on any one of them in the middle of the night and they would come.

I have a friend who has been on a spiritual search. He hasn't found the answers as yet but says he is a better person for trying. Praying has the same effect. When we pray for ourselves and others, something good happens.

I meditate every morning without fail. If I have an early appointment, I get up earlier so I can spend at least 45 minutes of inspirational reading and praying. I cannot start my day without this quiet time. First, you must clear your mind completely; make it a total blank. This is difficult at first because your mind keeps wandering, but with practice it becomes easier.

I have found that what works for me is a prayer book. At the top of the book it says, *I give all these concerns to God. Let go—let God and I promise not to take them back.* I write down every prayer for myself and others and also include prayers of gratitude. So often our prayers are asking and we should not forget to say thank you for our blessings. As I go over these prayers each day, I write down the answers, sometimes yes and sometimes no. My devotionals usually come from some inspirational book. By the time I finish, I am ready to meet the new day with joy. I sometimes say, "Something good is going to happen today" and it usually does.

At this point, you may want to tell me that what I say is all well and good but it does not apply to you. You would say that you have many worries, that your life is miserable and it's impossible to be happy. First, I would assume you want to be happy, but I guess there are people who enjoy being miserable although I cannot imagine why.

If you honestly would like to learn how to overcome worrying and being anxious all the time, perhaps you could try something that helped me. Get a piece of paper and on one side write *I HAVE NO CONTROL OVER.* Then list the things you are worrying about where you cannot affect the outcome. These might be issues about your children, grandchildren, other family members or friends. No one is asking your advice, but you are concerned. There really does come a time when your adult children make their own decisions without your impute. Actually, that is exactly what you hoped for when you were raising them. So what do you do? You pray about them and release them. In time, it becomes a habit to examine each issue that comes to mind. If you are not part of the solution, release it.

On the other side of the paper write *I DO HAVE CONTROL OVER* and list the items I need to work on. My list contains such things as patience, loving without judging and giving more of myself, resources and talents to others.

I have had people tell me that it sounds good, but how do you really release your anxieties. They will tell me that they cannot do that; that no matter how hard they try, those unwanted thoughts come back. Of course you have to have a real desire to want to think more positively. If you do, try this. During your daily activities, when you find unwanted thoughts coming into your mind, STOP, and say to yourself, "I release that concern to my God or Higher Power." Another thing I have learned is that so many things we worry about never happen. We have spent a great deal of time being anxious for no good reason. Releasing anxiety is not easy in the beginning, but the rewards are enormous.

Most of the cancer patients I have known are better people because of this traumatic experience. In time, I came to believe that being told you have cancer is a wake up call. It forces us to face our mortality and evaluate our lives and relationships. It teaches us to appreciate every day and every moment and it gives us more empathy and compassion for the suffering of others. The people I know who have been confronted with a life threatening disease are loving and forgiving. Perhaps it's because they have come to realize that life is too short to worry about real or imagined hurts. Many cancer patients, including myself, will tell you that cancer has enriched their lives.

How stress negatively effects our body has been the subject of many scientific studies. An article in the Chicago Tribune by Bob Condor cites a Dutch study at Vrije Univertiteit in Amsterdam that measures the effect of stress on the body. They found that over-commitment to work can impair the body's natural ability to dissolve blood clots, putting individuals at higher risk for heart disease.

Transcendental meditation, a structured form of practicing relaxation, was used in this research. The researchers found that in addition to meditation and physical activity, massage therapy and social support were other options for relieving stress. Some people seem to be optimistic by nature, but thinking positively is not easy for many others.

The study used a technique they called "focusing" on key parts of the body. The purpose was to increase awareness of how the mind and body affect each other. All of us have experienced the physical effects of the emotions of fear, anger, hate, love and joy. There is a sudden rush of adrenaline that floods our body. We do not live in a vacuum and we certainly cannot eliminate stress. We just need to learn how to eliminate the hurtful stress in order to lead healthier and happier lives.

Chapter IX

The Healing Power of Prayer

Is it fact or fiction?

In any discussion of the healing power of prayer, we have to deal with those people, both doctors and patients, who believe that prayer has no place in the practice of medicine. For those of you who depend on prayer to help you through life's difficulties, nothing is going to dissuade you of its benefits. The skeptics, on the other hand, want solid, concrete scientific evidence that it works. It is difficult to conduct controlled studies of the benefits of prayer to an individual's health, but there are some studies that are impressive.

Perhaps you have heard of Larry Dossey, M.D. He practiced medicine for many years using a strictly conventional approach. He considered himself to be what he called a "scientific" physician, but something was missing. He tells us that he grew up in a church but became an agnostic in college. After medical school and the Vietnam War, he became interested in the philosophies of the East, particularly Buddhism and Taoism. There came a time when he felt drawn to pray for his patients and eventually with them if they requested him to do so. He was amazed at the improvement in their health. Their mental attitude improved, they were calmer and, in some instances, the healings were miraculous.

This became such a compelling issue for Dossey that he has devoted the rest of his life to proving scientifically that prayer, indeed, does contribute to the healing process. Dossey says, "To be sure, prayer does not need science to legitimize or justify it. Even so, I believe that science *can* demonstrate the potency of prayer. People who pray are likely to feel empowered and validated in their beliefs as a result." This doctor has never suggested abandoning medical care but rather believes a complementary approach using both prayer and medical intervention produces the best possible results for the patient.

Dr. Dossey has written several books on this subject and cites scientific studies that use as much control as possible. He learned through his research that there have been over one hundred scientific studies on the power of prayer. They have proven that patients who pray or are prayed for do better then those who do not have the benefit of prayer.

Double blind studies have been used where patients with similar problems and treatments are divided into two groups—one group being prayed for, the other not. Neither the patients or the doctors knew which patients were in what group. Statistically, the ones being prayed for did better physically.

One interesting study Dossey explains is on interpersonal imagery. This is the ability of an image held by one person to make a difference in another person's body. In his book, *Healing Words and The Healing Power of Prayer* he cites the work of Dr. William Braud on this phenomenon. In a series of experiments, Braud, in collaboration with colleagues, has shown that the mental images of one person can modify the activity of the autonomic nervous system of a distant person. We know this as intercessory prayer.

Dr. Dale A. Matthew, an associate professor of medicine at Georgetown University School of Medicine, has compiled a large body of data about the effect of faith on physical healing. In addition, after years of observing his patients he concludes that those who pray have better results in overcoming illness.

An article in Forbes magazine, March 23, 1998, tells us the story of John Templeton, a retired mutual fund manager, who has dedicated his considerable fortune to scientific research in this field through his Foundation. Among other things, he funds research designed to measure the medical benefits of a spiritual lifestyle. There have been favorable studies at Duke University by Dr. Harold Koenig, at Dartmouth Medical School and at the UCLA School of Public Health.

A recently published book, *Seniors Guide to Pain-Free Living: All Natural Drug-Free Relief for Everything That Hurts* by Doug Dollemore and the editors of Prevention magazine devotes a chapter to the power of prayer in reducing pain.

The author cites evidence from many studies that suggest that prayer can have beneficial effects on nearly every system in the body, and especially the parts of the brain that regulate pain. According to this book, prayer is similar to relaxation techniques that elevate your mood, lower your blood pressure and heart rate, and relieve muscle tension. Prayer eases anxiety, depression, and other emotions that can intensify pain.

Dollemore does not say that prayer alone is going to cure chronic pain, but does believe it produces positive results if used with other techniques described in this book. I might add that there are many documented cases where patients ascribe their healing to the power of prayer.

Of course, those of us who already believe in the therapeutic benefit of prayer do not need studies to convince us. However, it is encouraging to know that there are some in the medical profession who are discovering the benefits of prayer.

I didn't know how to pray for a long time. In the back of my mind there was always a nagging doubt and it went something like this. "Why would God listen to anyone as insignificant as me about my concerns?" Also, when I prayed, it was more of a begging or complaining. Over time, I learned to pray differently. I still pray for many people every day—always to keep family and friends in His care. Sometimes, I have more specific prayers for those with cancer and other illnesses, those who are mourning the loss of a loved one, those who are in need of the means to provide for themselves and loved ones, and anyone who is going through difficult times. I name all these concerns, but then I release them to God (or Higher Power) for resolution. I have learned that my constant worry about a problem does not solve anything. In fact, it may affect my health. God does a much better job of taking care of His people then I ever did.

My prayer time would not be complete without prayers of gratitude for many blessings. When something you have diligently prayed for has been answered, do you say, "Thank You?" When a prayer is not answered as you would have wished, have you been able to say, "Your will be done, God?" I am sure you have heard the saying, "Be careful what you pray for, you might get it." I believe that there are times when God has something better in mind for us then what we think we desire. Have you ever looked back on your life and realized this? I have.

I am fortunate that I now have the time in the morning for meditation. In years past, when I had a large family to wake up, feed and get off to work and school, I could not manage that. It is wonderful to start the day with prayer and meditation, but we can pray anytime; driving to work, riding the bus and carpooling, for example. I used to become irritated when I had to wait in line for some service. Now I look at it as an opportunity to pray.

I think we are getting messages all the time if we really listen. I used to think it was intuition or coincidence. Often a name pops into my mind of a person I haven't been in contact with for sometime. I act on that now by writing or calling and nine times out of ten the other person will say, "I was just thinking about you." If we're going to ask God for direction or answers, we need to find time to listen.

I recently came across a wonderful book at the library with the title *The Healing Path of Prayer* by Ron Roth with Peter Occhiogrosso. The author was a Catholic priest for twenty-five years and now works full time teaching modern mysticism and healing through prayer to people of all faiths. This man never sought the power of healing, but believes it was a gift from God and that we all have the same power if we really open ourselves to the light and energy of God. He says that God expected all of us to have the same ability as Jesus possessed and cites Mark 11:24, "Therefore I tell you, whatever you ask for in prayer, believe that you have received it, and it will be yours." (From the NIV Study Bible)

There are many helpful suggestions in this book about prayer. Many of the words reinforced what I already believe and others gave me new insights on how to be a better prayer. The author suggests new ways to tap into the healing energy of God; not only physical healing but emotional and spiritual. I think we often put such importance on being strong. The author tells us that we receive the greatest gifts when we realize our own helplessness and dependency on God. That happened to me and has made such a difference in my life.

When I was diagnosed with cancer the second time, I was searching desperately for a release from fear and peace of mind. I went to hear a visiting minister speak. His name was Howard Thurman and he had a long list of credentials in the field of religion that I have listed elsewhere in this book. Never in my life have I encountered such a spiritual person. He had a radiance about him that is hard to describe.

Thurman's sermon was inspiring and on the way out from his lecture I bought several of his books. One of them, *Disciplines of the Spirit*, answered so many of my questions about faith. In fact, this little book led to my day of prayer and the surrender of my ego to God. I have never realized such peace as when I finally realized that I was not alone.

In this book, there is a chapter on prayer and in it Dr. Thurman describes the void so many of us feel as "the hunger of the heart." He believes that the experience of prayer, with practice, can be nurtured and cultivated. It is not hard to believe that for this man communion with God is as natural as eating and sleeping.

He talks about the structure of nature and how we are all part of that. Nature has always been a part of what convinces me that there is a God. When I look around me at the beauty and orderliness of this world, the predictability of the seasons that come and go right on schedule, it convinces me that there is a divine plan.

The author wonders how man can investigate the external world, recognize its order, declare that there are certain generalities about its behavior which he calls laws. Then man can study the organism called man and discover a certain orderliness of inner behavior and yet think of man as an entity apart from the rest of creation. Thurman believes that "man is body. But more than body: mind, but more than mind: feelings, but more than feelings. Man is total; moreover, he is spirit." And it is this spirit that connects him with the Creator of Life.

There is a harmony in nature and between man and God. In recognizing this, man opens up the lines of communication between himself and the Creator of all things. The author says, "The true purpose of all spiritual disciplines is to clear away whatever may block that which is God in us" and he emphasizes the importance of silence. He tells us that silence is attained in many ways and that each person finds that in his own way. It is necessary in order to attain a calmness, to eliminate distractions and to find that connection with a Higher Power.

I found it illuminating that Thurman speaks of the benefits to ourselves when praying for others and also the benefits of prayers of thanksgiving. I have found that it is hard to be depressed when I'm counting my blessings.

Have you ever had any miracles in your life? When I look back over my life, I believe that divine intervention is the only possible answer. One of the most frightening times of my life was when our five year old son, Jim, had polio. He had been ill for about a week with a fever. He was listless and was having difficulty eating.

In those days before the polio vaccine, the summer months were a frightening time because that is when the epidemics of polio seemed to occur. Every year we would usually hear of some friend who had contracted this dreaded disease.

Our pediatrician came to see Jim every afternoon and I noticed he was testing his reflexes. Finally, one day he couldn't swallow at all and the doctor said we had to get him to the hospital. I heard him say "bulbar" and my heart practically stopped. At the hospital when they were wheeling him off to do a spinal tap, it was almost more then I could bear. This could not be happening to this sweet child with blond curly hair and big blue eyes.

There are three kinds of polio and bulbar is the worst because as it progresses it paralyzes the lungs and the patient has to be placed in an iron lung to keep him breathing. Jim was in isolation because of the infectious nature of the disease, he couldn't swallow, and someone had to keep suctioning the saliva out of his mouth and throat or he would have choked to death. His Dad spent hours by his beside keeping his throat clear. The iron lung was waiting outside the door for him. There was no treatment for polio. It was just allowed to run its course. With Jim, it stopped before it reached his lungs and he came home.

The only after effects he had were weakened throat and abdominal muscles. Because of the weakness of his abdominal muscles, he would get epidemic vomiting. I used to spend whole days giving him a teaspoon of water every fifteen minutes. He would keep it down for an hour or so and then start vomiting again. He would get so dehydrated that he would have to be given intravenous fluids. He gradually recovered and in a year or two he was completely well.

Today, many years later, he is a very healthy, productive adult with a wife and two children. He is a mountaineer, a skier and is very active in his community especially in issues that involve children. Almost every time I look at him, I thank God. And, yes, I do think it was a miracle that he was spared the devastating effects of polio.

There are many other instances in my life when I now feel God was watching over me and my family. I was not always with God, but *He was always with me.*

The thing about faith is that each of has to find his own way. For many years because I felt a void in my life and I truly wanted to believe, I read many books on religion and asked many questions of both lay people and clergy. I know now that I do not have to have the answers to all those questions. Some things are simply beyond our understanding. When the light finally came, it was faith given to me by the grace of God not because I ever did anything to earn it. I still don't have the answers to all my questions but it doesn't seem to matter anymore. What matters is that I feel a presence all around me and a love beyond understanding.

Chapter X

Support Groups

I consider myself privileged to have been involved with an incredible support group. It was started about fifteen years ago by a cancer patient and meets every Wednesday evening the year around. It has never been advertised. Patients hear about the positive results of this group from friends and today there are anywhere from thirty-five to fifty who attend. Cancer patients, their families and friends come together every week to share where they are on the road to recovery and what they are doing mentally, physically and emotionally to attain good health.

These people have taken charge of their lives and want to learn everything possible that will help them back to wellness. As stories are shared, there is no criticism of treatment chosen. Rather, each person is supported in an understanding and loving way. It is amazing at the bond that is formed in a group where everyone is focused on a common enemy. In this case, cancer.

This group was formed many years after my initial battle with cancer. How I wish it had been available when I was going through the early stages and treatment of this disease. I was pretty much alone as I struggled to get control of my illness and myself. As I look back, what I did was beneficial. I read many books. Some to help me learn more about the disease and many others were inspirational books. It helped me to read success stories. Farther on in this book I have compiled a list of books with a short synopsis for each.

I heard about the support group shortly after it began and decided to attend to see if I could help and I eventually became the facilitator. I went primarily to see if sharing my experience would help anyone just beginning this process. As it usually happens, I gained far more from this courageous group then I ever gave. Listening to their remarkable stories week after week was so inspirational. I also formed some wonderful and long lasting friendships over the years.

There was Alice (name changed) who had been diagnosed with Stage IV ovarian cancer. After her surgery at a local hospital, she and her husband were told she had six weeks to two months to live. Even with this prognosis, they recommended chemotherapy. Her husband contacted me through mutual friends and we met for dinner. He was in a panic and frantic to know what, if anything, to do. I explained the success of my treatment with immunotherapy and he immediately transferred Alice into the care of my doctor. That was the day she started on the road to recovery and she is still living many years later. Alice came to support group to tell her success story and encourage others with a similar problem.

Then there was Mary (name changed) who had surgery for breast cancer and eighteen out of twenty-five lymph nodes showed cancer involvement. I had never heard of anyone who had that many affected lymph nodes and certainly her prognosis was not good. Her disease would almost certainly metastasize (spread) to other areas of her body. Her doctor recommended chemotherapy but without much enthusiasm. Mary also chose another doctor and immunotherapy and is a long time survivor with no spread of cancer. She has been coming to support group faithfully for years and has taken voluminous notes. If anyone wants to know what happened five years ago, all they have to do is ask

Mary to look it up in her notebook. I guess you could say she is the historian of the group.

The group of men who have (or have had) prostate cancer usually sit together. None of them have had surgery. Most of them are on hormone therapy in addition to other changes they have made in their lifestyles. They have various theories on why they have done well. One member of the group is sure that the fact that he juiced fifty pounds of carrots a week was responsible for his recovery. Others have increased their exercise program, taken courses in meditation and/or relaxation techniques. Everyone is anxious to share what he or she believe helped in their recovery. This group meets for lunch once a month in addition to attending support group every week.

We had a gentleman who was depressed and negative. Every week he had a litany of complaints about his health and life in general. Everyone tried so hard to help him have a more positive attitude. He quit coming after awhile. I think he was afraid we might cheer him up and he really did want to wallow in his misery. However, most of the people who come each week are honestly seeking not only information on treatment, but help to overcome their fears and anxieties.

What did we talk about? In the beginning, when the group was smaller, we sat in a circle and everyone had an opportunity to talk about himself; his progress, his concerns and fears. No one was required to share and could pass when their turn came. I believe the uniqueness of this group was due to the fact that longtime survivors attended to help others who were going through the beginning stages of this frightening disease.

A young girl came up to me after our meeting one evening and said, "This is the one year anniversary of my diagnosis of breast cancer. I want to thank you because I couldn't have done it without you." I was amazed as I could not recall doing anything special for her and told her so. She replied, "You helped me because you were here. Every time I looked at you I thought, if she could do it, so can I."

The people in this group were remarkably upbeat. Sometimes there were tears, but more often there was a positive feeling of hope and even laughter as they shared their sometimes bizarre experiences. A camaraderie developed that was loving and lasting. They talked about everything they were doing: such as, juicing and what kind of processor to buy, diets, exercise, positive attitudes and spiritual renewal. They shared and applauded every success of the members. I always came away from these meetings feeling renewed. There were fun times, too, where everyone gathered for potlucks.

I have been told that some support groups are depressing because there is too much emphasis on dying. Our group emphasized living. We lost people, of course, and that was very sad, but we were able to be there for the families. It is true that each of us is going to die sometime, but until that time we need to live each day to the fullest. Someone asked me recently if I wasn't afraid of dying. My response was that I had decided that getting up each morning worrying about how long I was going to live probably was not going to help me to live one day longer. So, I just try to embrace each day with joy.

I would strongly urge you to find a support group that fits your needs. If you cannot find one, start one with a few cancer patients. If you are going to meet in your church, put a note on the bulletin board or in your church newsletter. Perhaps your doctor will allow you to put a notice in his waiting room. Word of mouth will bring others to your meetings.

Chapter XI

Passion for Living

How do we live our lives with joy regardless of our circumstances? It has to do with realizing we are not alone in this journey through life. It is finding an inner resource that sustains us when times are tough. It is a belief that even though today is bad, tomorrow will be better. We may never completely get over deep sorrows, but we can learn to accept them and go on.

Life does not always seem fair. Sometimes we feel that we are literally bombarded with loss, tragedy, illness, financial problems or just the difficulty of getting through each day with grace and good humor. I believe that it is not the things that happen to us, but how we react to the unfolding events in our lives that make the difference. Certainly, it's hard to be thankful when bad things happen to us, but, with God's grace, we can cope. There are countless examples of people who have worked to make some good come out of the tragedy in their lives.

Tragedy changes your life forever and I have enormous admiration for those persons who somehow manage to rise above all the pain and make their lives count. There are events such as losing a child or becoming physically disabled that are beyond our comprehension. Years ago, when I was in college, a good friend, Elliot, (name changed) only eighteen years old, was paralyzed in an automobile accident. He was a tall, handsome guy and a member of the nationally recognized crew at our university. Elliot was told he would never walk again. He went into a deep depression and had no will to live.

Several years after this dreadful event, Elliot's family sent him to a rehabilitation center in California. They were hopeful that he could learn to walk with braces. While there he met Margaret (name changed) who had been paralyzed in a similar accident when she was only sixteen years old. They fell in love and although they spent most of their time in wheelchairs, with the assistance of braces they did walk down the aisle when they were married.

Margaret transformed Elliot's life and from that time on, their lives were filled with joy. They were an inspiration to everyone who knew them. Elliot worked in the family business and they owned their own home. They entertained, went to football games and other activities. They had a hand driven car and took trips. One time I asked Elliot what happened if they had a flat tire or some other mechanical difficulty. He said, "Well, we just put on our flashing lights and wait until someone stops to help us."

They felt so fortunate to have each other and the resources to live a comfortable life that they tried to help others who were handicapped. Elliot started a program for wheelchair athletes and also an organization to provide wheelchairs to those in need. Both of them had a passion for living and they were fun to be with. I am sure there were private moments of sadness over what had happened to them, but they made the most of what they had left.

How do we get to a place where there is happiness in our lives? My solutions will probably not be the same as yours. I am hopeful, though, that they may give you some insight on where to begin.

REACHING OUT TO OTHERS—Nothing pulls me out of self pity faster than helping someone else in need. When I do this, I don't have time to feel sorry for myself. Visit a sick friend or take a lonely person out to lunch or dinner. If you volunteer at a shelter for the homeless, you cannot help being grateful that you have a place to live. If you volunteer at an emergency feeding program, you will be grateful that you have enough to eat. The opportunities for volunteering are limitless: visiting prisons, building houses for Habitat for Humanity, coaching youth sports teams, giving rides to the housebound, tutoring students, teaching adults to read are some of the things you could do.

My son does volunteer work for a DayCare Center that takes care of homeless pre-school children. He has a card with the following wonderful quotation. The title is PRIORITIES and it reads, "A hundred years from now it will not matter what my bank account was, the sort of house I lived in, or the kind of car I drove…but the world may be different because I was important in the life of a child."

When we reach out to others, initially we are thinking only about giving, but usually we receive so much more then we give. It also gives us a plan for our daily living and makes us feel good about ourselves. You might have to try several different things before you find the right fit for you. Whatever it is, it needs to be something you really enjoy and that you look forward to doing and can embrace with enthusiasm and passion.

We will probably never know how our helping hand affects the lives of others. Yet, it is hard to imagine a community without volunteers. They are the glue that makes it work.

It took me a long time to learn that it's OK to say NO. We have no choice in certain responsibilities such as taking care of our families. However, we do have control over our outside activities and we need to learn how to manage our time. There is nothing to be gained by overloading our schedule. In fact, it just adds more stress to our lives. So, we need to find a balance and say YES to the things that we feel will enrich us and give us a sense of accomplishment.

One way to accomplish this is to make a list of priorities and stick to it. If you feel pressured to say YES when you want to say NO, ask the person requesting your time if you can call her back the next day. By then, you can come up with an adequate response. You really do not need to explain or feel guilty. It's your life and only you know which activities you can assume with enthusiasm. When someone asks you to take on some project that you either do not have time for, is beyond your expertise or simply does not interest you, it's all right to say, "Thank you for asking me, but I am unable to do that at this time."

One thing I have learned is that if I overload my schedule, I don't do any one thing very well. Instead of feeling good about my life, I feel frantic, tired and pushed because I have left little or no time for myself.

I need to be involved in activities and causes that I feel passionate about. Because I feel so blessed that I have survived cancer for so many years, I feel passionate about wanting to help other cancer patients. I need to keep my schedule flexible so that I am available when people need me. I have a deep commitment to and involvement in my church. I am constantly resetting my goals and listening for direction from that inner voice. I strive for the balance in my life between activities and the quiet time I need to replenish my soul.

HAVING FUN—Making time just to be with the people I love is very important to me. I need to make time for being with friends and family who make me happy and make me laugh. I really do not know how anyone gets through life without a sense of humor. We even need to laugh at ourselves sometimes and not take everything so seriously.

Having fun for me includes lunch or dinner with friends or family, sporting events, enjoying a play or movie or just being with another person who lifts me up. When my husband died and I was alone for the first time in my life, many people asked me to do things. At first, my inclination was to say no. I didn't feel ready to face the world by myself. On the other hand, I thought if I refused invitations, I might not be asked again. So usually I went and there were times when I wondered why I was there, but mostly it was a good thing. We need to socialize, to get into the mainstream of life instead of nurturing our grief.

Another thing I have learned, especially since I've been alone, is not to expect others always to do for me. In other words, I try to reciprocate for all the goodness that is expressed to me.

ATTITUDE—Do we go through life as a victim always expecting the worst? Or do we greet each day as a new beginning; a day full of possibilities? I cannot say it better than a quotation from Charles Swindohl: "The longer I live, the more I realize the impact of attitude on life. Attitude, to me, is more important than the past, than education, than money, than circumstances, than failure, than successes, than what other people think or say or do. It is more important than appearance, giftedness, or skill. It will make or break a company—a church—a home. The remarkable thing is we have a choice every day regarding the attitude we will embrace for that day. We cannot change our past—we cannot change the fact that people will act a certain way. We cannot change the inevitable. The only thing we can do is play on the one string we have, and that is our attitude—I am convinced that life is 10% what happens to me and 90% how I react to it. And so it is with you—we are in charge of our Attitude."

LOVING—In the first place, I cannot accept the love offered to me if I am unable to love myself. I need to feel that I am a good person, certainly not perfect and prone to mistakes, but, still, someone who tries to be loving and helpful to others.

Unconditional love is the key, I believe, to loving and being loved. I don't quit loving others because they sometimes disappoint me. Instead, I try to realize that they must be trying to work through their own problems and perhaps if I love them even more, it will help. It is easy to love the lovable; loving those who are, at the moment, unlovable is more difficult,

It is hard for me to understand people who are bored without much purpose in life because every day is a gift and we can choose how we want to live. Of course there are no possibilities if we sit around feeling sorry for ourselves. Praying for direction and then taking action is necessary.

Chapter XII

Other Life Situations

The coping skills I learned in dealing with my cancer helped me with other crisis situations in my life.

Shortly after I was diagnosed with breast cancer, my husband, Ben, began having angina pain and after numerous tests it was determined that he had a blocked artery. By-pass surgery was recommended. This was a relatively new procedure at that time with considerable risks. I called my surgeon for advice and he told me not to go ahead without bringing in another heart specialist to review all the tests. This outside doctor concurred that by-pass surgery was his only option if he was going to survive. There was even a discussion of taking him to a hospital back East where more successful by-pass surgeries had been completed. However, it was decided that he was too critically ill to move so I, along with Ben and our family, made the decision to go ahead with the operation.

Ben was one of the early recipients of this operation in this area and the aftermath was excruciatingly painful. Thankfully, much improvement has been made in how this operation is performed since then because there would come a time when he would need a second by-pass surgery.

Ben's recovery was slow, but he did regain his health and went back to work. He remarked at the time that he would never go through that operation again. I had survived breast cancer, he had survived a serious heart problem, and we were grateful. There certainly were emotional, stressful ups and downs during this time, but you get through it somehow.

Our children were twenty-four, twenty-two, twenty and thirteen at the time. Years later the youngest told me that I failed to talk to her enough and that she was frightened all the time that one or both of us were going to die. I thought I was being completely honest with the children, but apparently I did not communicate well enough and I regret that. I do know that neither Ben nor I thought we were going to die. I realize, however, that when you have a life threatening illness you are so consumed with your own problems that you often don't relate very well to the real world.

Several normal years went by before everything fell apart again. My cancer had metastasized to the bone and shortly after that bad news, Ben was diagnosed with bladder cancer. It was then that my life turned around in a big way. The spiritual experience I had at that time took all my fear away and I began to address other changes I needed to make in my life.

I had begun my treatment with immunotherapy and Ben was treated by the same doctor. We were both receiving BCG. I believe Ben was one of the first bladder cancer patients to receive BCG directly into the bladder. He used to go to the doctor on his way home from work. He never had any side effects and his cancer was under control for sixteen years when he died of heart problems. Today BCG is the treatment of choice for bladder cancer. I think often of how many patients could have benefited during all the years it was considered experimental.

There were months and years of appointments and tests with doctors for both of us and other times when everything was fairly normal.

Then, nine years after Ben had his first by-pass, he was having angina pain again. He never talked or complained much about his health. That was never more apparent than when I was having a leisurely cup of coffee one morning. Ben was dressed and ready to go to work. On his way out he said, "I'm having chest pains and I'm going to stop at the hospital on my way to work." I asked him to wait until I could get dressed and go with him.

He never did get to work that day or for sometime afterward. Tests showed that the same artery was blocked again. His surgeon told us that he could not operate because there was nothing left to by-pass. Both of us have had many wonderful, caring doctors, but this surgeon was so arrogant that I wanted to move him to another hospital. However, Ben was in critical condition and in terrible pain so that was not possible. In fact, he was dying. So I asked for an outside review and this doctor disagreed with the first doctor and said that, in his opinion, there was a possibility that a second by-pass would be successful. It was decided to go ahead and try. There really was not any other choice and Ben agreed to go through the operation for the second time.

Even so, it was unsettling to have a surgeon operating on your husband when he was firmly convinced that there was no chance for success. This surgeon complained that he was overruled by committee, that it would take him two and a half hours to even get to the bypass area and then he wouldn't be able to do anything. However, he was nice enough to send word out from the operating room that he was wrong. That surgery gave Ben nine more years.

My experiences have shown me that every patient needs an advocate. Whether it is a family member, friend or pastor, it is absolutely essential. When you are too sick to fight for yourself, you need someone asking questions and demanding answers.

While I was battling for Ben's life, I had an episode that shows what stress can do. I had arrived at the hospital and my heart was beating really hard. I thought it would stop, but it was still wildly irregular while

I visited with him and then as I sat in the waiting room. Finally, I went to the nurse's station and asked if I could lie down somewhere. That was a mistake as the next thing I knew I was in emergency and ended up in the Coronary Care Unit with Ben. Now our children had to deal with both parents in a critical care unit. While I was in emergency, my youngest daughter appeared at my side. I said, "How did you know about this situation so quickly?" She replied, "I just came down to the hospital to have lunch with you and they said, 'Your Mother is in emergency.'"

I know that this episode resulted from stress because I did not then, nor any time since, have a heart problem. I have never had any episodes of irregular heart beat since I learned how to handle stressful situations. Sometimes life simply overwhelms us and those are the times when we need to call on every resource available. Don't be afraid to ask for help. One of my problems has been always thinking that I can handle everything by myself.

There were good times in between our crisis situations. I find that when I am confronted with life threatening situations and survive, I breathe a sigh of relief, say thank you and go on. We didn't dwell on our health problems and perhaps that is the reason we didn't share enough with our children.

Ben died of heart related problems nine years after his second by-pass surgery. Even with all the previous crises, it was quite sudden and unexpected. I had lived at home until I was married so I had never experienced living alone. I am not going to tell you that I was never sad or lonely because that would not be true. It was a big adjustment and a new challenge.

When the initial shock was over, I did some serious thinking about what I had left to live for. When I counted my blessings, I had many. I had a beautiful home, financial security and my health. I was surrounded by loving, caring family and friends and I was involved in activities that were meaningful and productive. I realized that even though I did not choose to be alone, it was the first time since I was thirteen that I was not responsible for anyone but myself. This presented an opportunity to do things I had never been able to fit into a busy schedule.

Happiness is a choice and I chose to be happy with the blessings that were left to me. All of my children and grandchildren are wonderful and loving, but I do not expect them to fill up my life. In fact, I don't just sit around waiting for something to happen. I make it happen. This precious life is too good to waste feeling sorry for myself.

Chapter XIII

What Can We Do about Pain?

A discussion of pain is a difficult subject because there are many degrees of pain. Our ability to tolerate pain is different and our experiences vary.

Acute pain is a signal to the body that it has been damaged in some way. It is any physical pain with a discernible cause. A simple example would be hitting your thumb with a hammer. *Chronic* pain is persistent and constant. It may be in just one specific area or it may be the kind of pain that manifests itself in many areas of the body.

Pain that we know is temporary from surgery or an injury can be dealt with effectively with pain medication. However, long term use of medications is not advisable nor does it solve the problem. I have had pain of varying intensity over the years so I can speak from experience.

Years ago I had excruciating pain from a disc that slipped in and out in the lower part of my back. There would be long periods when I was pain free. Then, there came a time when it became so bad that I had trouble functioning. I know what it's like to get up in the morning wondering how I would get through the day. I did take pain medications at that time when the pain became unbearable. However, they were a mixed blessing because although they lessened the pain they made me feel sluggish and depressed and they did not solve the problem

X-rays did not reveal what was causing the pain so my doctor tried everything. I wore a brace, went to an osteopath and even had traction in the hospital in an attempt to realign my spine. Nothing worked and I finally had a myelogram. This is a procedure where the spinal fluid is withdrawn and a dye is injected into the spine. An x-ray film showed that the disc had ruptured and the pieces were pressing on the nerves in my lower back. Successful surgery was performed, my spine was fused to my tailbone with screws and I was finally pain free. So in this case, medical intervention solved my problem.

Another time I was rear-ended in an automobile accident that resulted in pain in my head and down my arm. Medical tests showed that I had a partially herniated disc in my neck and a bone chip. The neurosurgeon wanted to operate and told me terrible things that could happen if I did not have surgery. One of the things I remember distinctly is that he said I could become paralyzed. My decision was not to risk surgery without trying other things. This was what I call manageable pain because it didn't incapacitate me, but it was persistent.

After going to several physical therapists that were not able to help me, I found a therapist who practiced myofacial therapy which is a different kind of procedure. The therapist finds and uses trigger points in the body to effect healing. It was amazingly effective for me.

I feel very fortunate not to have had much pain with my cancer. I experienced a brief period of pain and discomfort from the radical mastectomy after my breast cancer, but had none with the bone cancer. My oncologist did not believe me at first and said it would be difficult to treat me if I minimized my pain. I did finally convince him that except for a sharp twinge once in awhile I was really pain free. I attribute this to my mental attitude and the fact that through spiritual intervention I had no fear. Due to the lack of pain and the fact that my treatment had no side effects, I came through my cancer experience feeling very well.

Other cancer patients are not so fortunate and the ones I have been privileged to know learned to deal with their pain in many ways. They were neither passive nor long-suffering patients. They tried many different things such as, acupuncture, relaxation techniques, biofeedback, exercise, and, for many, the power of prayer. They also went to a support group to learn about what worked for other patients. The camaraderie in that group helped tremendously with the mental attitude of the patients who attended. It really helps to know that you are not alone.

Chronic pain is a different problem altogether. An experience I had with pain about a year and a half ago gave me a new respect for people whose pain is unrelenting and unending. I had been in very good health for many years when I had a sudden onset of pain all over my body. It was in my arms, hands, shoulders, hips and legs. I cannot tolerate most pain medications so I had very little relief. It was like being healthy one day and an invalid the next. It began in October and by January I was in a wheelchair because the pain was so severe I couldn't walk. My doctor was as mystified as I was until a specialist diagnosed my problem as PMR (Polymyalgia Rheumatica). I don't know whether that diagnosis was correct, but I reluctantly agreed to take a low dose of prednisone. I say 'reluctantly' because I do not like to take drugs and I also knew that there were possible side effects from this one. I believe this helped, but it still doesn't explain why the pain was completely gone in the next two months. I used the wheelchair for just three weeks, then a cane and finally the day came that I could say I was pain free.

I prayed a lot for healing and I believe those prayers were answered. It was a humbling experience and it gave me a new respect for people who have chronic pain. We need to learn something from every experience in our lives and I think I did. Why did it happen? I don't know, but recovering from that episode of pain gave me a renewed appreciation for my life and filled me with joy.

I cannot even imagine the agony of being in pain every day of one's life. I recently read a book *The Chronic Pain Workbook* by Ellen Mohr

Catalano, M.A. that explains that this type of pain is seldom cured. Rather, the patient must learn to control the pain rather then let it control him. Chronic pain affects every aspect of the patient's life. Often the person suffering such pain feels that family and friends do not understand. Family and work relationships suffer and this, in turn, causes depression. The author believes new strategies involve working with the *whole* person and not just the symptoms. Pills are replaced with skills such as stress management, self-hypnosis, biofeedback, exercise; anything that brings about relaxation. When you are in constant pain, your whole body is tense and that causes more pain.

The best book I have read on this subject is *Chronic Pain: Taking Command of Our Healing* by Wm. R.B. Anderson, Ph.D. with Jesse F. Taylor, Ph.D. Anderson says, "Unfortunately, the Medical Establishment is slow to expand its range of theories in the search for effective treatments…while many doctors will, informally, admit that emotional effects are important in healing, they are hesitant to give professional credence to procedures which treat emotions in order to heal physical illness."

The authors believe that emotional trauma lies at the base of most chronic pain. The ideas presented in this book are not offered as an alternative to successful therapy. Rather, they are offered as an aid to hasten healing. Our belief systems collected over a lifetime are not arrived at consciously. In fact, many of them are buried deep in our subconscious mind. From my own experience, I know that treating just the disease is not enough. It is a joint effort between patient and doctor.

There have been extensive studies on endorphins and their role in controlling pain. Endorphins are chemicals secreted by the body that are natural painkillers. Production is unpredictable and not everyone produces the same amount of endorphins under each circumstance. It has been proven that stress and fear reduces the amount of this chemical that is produced. So, it would seem like common sense to work toward relieving the stress and fear in your life in an effort to boost your body's healing capabilities.

I talked to a friend who has been suffering with pain for years. His illness has been diagnosed as fibromyalgia or chronic myofacial pain syndrome. This is an incurable condition that produces pain in the fibrous muscle tissue. Over the years that he has been afflicted with this disease, he has tried almost everything that medical science and alternative medicine has to offer. The following is what he said in his search for healing. "My most severe chronic pain began in January, 1996 with pronounced pain at the end of my rib cage. I do not know what the trigger (or cause) for this onset of pain can be attributed to. Trauma, of one sort or another, has been mentioned in literature as a cause but some pain specialists discount this notion. I guess my initial painful episodes were the result of emotional stress.

"I was referred to a doctor who specializes in Rhuematology/ Osteoporosis/ and Fibromyalgia diagnosis and treatments. Main stream doctors are sympathetic if they have studied or been exposed to the new evidence and AMA diagnostic procedures.

"Through the years my symptoms and pain levels have varied. Conventional and non-traditional medicine have been used, none with much success. My treatments have included acupuncture, physical therapy, biofeedback, and some counseling. I have not gone to a pain clinic.

"I have attempted to resolve a personal problem by moving and living by myself. Since then, my stress level has been reduced and thus my pain levels and frequencies of flare periods have diminished greatly. I have stopped taking long term medications such as Nuerontin and Vioxx.

"I finally realized I had a drinking problem and am now in treatment. I do feel much better since I stopped drinking. However, as I write this I am in a flared condition with increased pain and I have no idea what triggered this episode. These episodes are much like the onset of the flu, but without the stomach distress, nausea or head cold symptoms. A lot of generalized pain in the muscles and joints is typical.

"Most of this condition, or a great deal of it, may be induced by weather changes or emotional stress. At least these two seem to affect me with regularity and predictable results."

One of my daughters had to have surgery for a suspicious growth on her ovary. The surgeon would not know until after the operation whether it was cancer or a benign cyst. She was very fortunate that it turned out to be the latter. The most remarkable thing, however, was how she handled the pain. Growing up she was very fearful of any kind of pain even if it was a minor thing like a shot.

She stayed with me after her surgery and I was amazed at how quickly she recovered with a minimum of pain. I asked her how she accomplished that and this is what she said: "Several things helped me deal with the pain of my surgery. I read Dr. Bernie Siegel's book *Love, Medicine and Miracles* and it gave me hope. I followed my oncologist's suggestions on getting in shape before the surgery, which helped me recover without any problems. I also was pretty good at following his instructions such as limitations after surgery. I think trusting my medical team (including nurses) was very important to me.

"Siegel's book suggested that I could ask the doctors to talk to me during surgery. It would be like hypnotic suggestion. I asked the anesthesiologist to talk to me about how I did not smoke and had no fear of pain. I had no compulsion to smoke after surgery and I had been afraid that would be a problem.

"While I was in the hospital, my surgeon lectured me because I was not taking the pain medication as regularly scheduled. My response to him was that was because I was in no pain.

"I have no doubt that for me a lot of previous pain was caused by fear. Clearly, when a person is afraid they tense up and, as a result, have more pain. Relaxing is part of the key. But to me, it was a miracle that this one suggestion during surgery took away the fear of pain for me and, as a result, the pain itself."

I asked a nurse friend to give me her observations on how pain is handled in a hospital setting by both nurses and doctors. She sees pain on a daily basis and this is what she said: "Almost without exception, the patients I deal with have pain at one point or another. Many discovered they were ill because the pain started and others have pain after they have surgery. As nurses, we assess the entire patient at the start of each shift, reviewing each system such as cardiovascular, respiratory, nutrition, etc., including a 'system' of comfort. We view comfort as an important part of the patient's well-being and over the past few years have focused on improving our assessment skills and also helping the patient identify and define their pain.

"We evaluate the location, duration, aggravating factors and intensity (scale of 0-no pain to 10-unbearable pain), so that as different staff tend to the patient, we have a more consistent process for evaluating the pain. That being said, the process for achieving acceptable patient comfort becomes a gray area because pain is very different to different people. Another system we assess is psychological and of course one's sense of self, loss of power over one's own body and one's experiences with pain in the past (his own or that observed) can all greatly influence one's perception of one's own pain.

"Although it may not be correct, the medical profession's general first line of offense against pain is medication. There are safe standards for pain medication doses and doctors generally order a range for the patient and have the nurse use her judgment on what may work for the patient, then adjust accordingly. I find that I assess the patient, taking in his information about his pain, then observe his non-verbal behavior as well as listen to his other concerns.

"Many times solving other concerns can decrease the pain level and thus require less medication, usually a narcotic. This is where the psychosocial aspect comes in, watching family interactions, observing the timing of the pain medication request (when the patient is alone, frightened) or even comparing or competing with a roommate. Two patients with similar surgeries and assumed similar pain can have very different levels of pain based on many of these factors. Something as simple as repositioning, changing temperature, backrubs, quiet, helping the patient understand the reason for the pain or staying a few extra minutes in the room can decrease the patient's pain. Yet, we as nurses are at times rushed and may find medication the most available and convenient answer. We are working on that!

"I think doctors try to keep their patients comfortable with medications, but when what they have ordered doesn't work, nurses often are the ones to suggest alternate medications, dosages, etc. and become the patient's advocate for comfort. Because we are with the patient so much more, we have a better sense of what else might work. Most doctors seem sensitive to the patient's discomfort, but don't feel the urgency for change since they are not with the patient.

"For chronic pain situations, there are Pain Clinics at most major medical centers to which doctors will refer difficult cases. I would say that these cases are considered troublesome by doctors (and many nurses) and we probably do not appreciate all the factors that are involved in the patient's pain and these types of patients get labeled as drug-dependent, psychologically weaker and imbalanced.

"This is an area we all need to work on. It is hard to empathize with a patient who says he is having horrible pain, yet is on immense amounts of drugs, far greater than most patients in similar circumstances would require, and often his non-verbal behavior does not demonstrate intense pain. We have to remember, however, that this type of patient has REAL PAIN within his own perception and he needs help dealing with it and overpowering it. This actually goes for all patients and their pain.

"Some patients do deal with pain better than others. One interesting observation that I have discovered is that elderly people seem to deal with pain in a more accepting manner. Men and women seem to deal about the same. The difference is mostly based on a person's personality, their own perception of what pain is all about, their sense of being part of their healing process and the support they have within the family circle."

The following comments are the observations of a caregiver. Although she has never been in pain except during childbirth, she has had to deal with pain in varying degrees of severity with her husband and children. She told me that she thinks pain is a very personal thing. Individuals seem to have different tolerances and handle it differently.

She feels that mind and emotions play a big part. She believes that control is a major issue. Being able to let go and know you are not in control of your life helps with getting rid of pain. In childbirth, learning how to relax is key, in her opinion. When she was delivering her first child, she remembers how the girl next to her screamed for hours until she finally asked the nurse if this person was going to have her baby soon. The nurse replied, "You are a lot farther along than she is."

Any of you who have children, has probably noticed that they have different tolerances to pain. I know I did. It seemed that one child didn't feel pain as acutely as another. This caregiver shares the reactions of her children. One would be hysterical with a slight injury while another would hardly react. She felt that in addition to the pain their emotional makeup was different.

When her husband became ill, it was a long time before he received a diagnosis of cancer, but he was in pain. He had severe headaches and went to a clinic that specializes in this disorder. They used biofeedback along with other techniques in an effort to get to the bottom of his stress level. The patient knew something was terribly wrong and it manifested itself in headaches and also painful backaches. What is interesting is that when he knew he had cancer the headaches and backaches disappeared.

This caregiver doesn't give doctors very high marks in dealing with a patient's pain. Their solution is just to give medicine without trying to find the cause. From her experience, she says it is important to take as little medication as possible in the beginning because long term, as you have to increase the dosage, it might not work as well. Doctors should be looking carefully for side effects and allergic reactions.

As the nurse stated, when pain is beyond the control of the doctor, he will often suggest going to a pain clinic. This caregiver feels that pain clinics, however, are only as good as the patient attending. If the patient doesn't listen and cooperate, they cannot be successful.

The most helpful role of the caregiver is to do research so she will be knowledgeable about her patient's illness and to be an advocate for that person. One of the things this caregiver mentioned was the need to be aggressive in reaching doctors; not allowing the patient to go too long without help. Also, it is important to monitor medicine intake and to encourage consistency. She found that if her husband skipped taking medications prescribed by his doctor, the consequences were serious.

As an advocate when her husband was in severe pain because she had done research, she was able to persuade his doctor to perform spinal nerve blocks. At the time, they were really helpful and necessary, but had never been suggested by the attending physician. She felt good about being the one able to get him this help.

When a member of the family has a serious illness, it is hard on everyone and the caregiver tries to keep a balance. In this particular instance, there were many months when the children could not have their friends come to their house because their father needed absolute quiet. The patient becomes the primary concern and everyone suffers to some degree.

Looking back, this particular caregiver said, "I guess what I would do differently is to be more sensitive and aware of what was going on. I would watch mood swings and language more. There is a lot of emotional pain associated with physical pain and if I had dealt more with the emotional pain, it could have helped the physical pain."

There are many natural remedies suggested for pain. If you are interested in exploring that possibility, I would suggest that you find books on that subject at your library. Since most natural products are harmless, there is no reason not to try them.

Chapter XIV

Reading List

These are my recommendations of books that I think will be helpful to any of you who are struggling to overcome cancer or any other difficulty you are having in your quest to leading a happy, healthful life. I believe that reading gives us inspiration and new insights. Also, it is often good to know that we are not the only ones who are searching for a better, more productive compassionate reason for living.

Love, Medicine and Miracles by Bernie Siegel, M.D. Published in 1986 this book was one of the early books to explore the connection between the body and the mind. It is the story of the author's own growth from an overworked surgeon with no joy in his chosen profession to a medical practitioner grateful for the dramatic changes in his life and the lives of his patients as he becomes involved in a loving, caring way with those he would heal. The book is full of concrete suggestions for a better, healthier life, some of which are: good nutrition, exercise, having fun, loving yourself and others, relaxation and meditation.

Peace, Love and Healing by Bernie Siegel, M.D. The doctor continues to explore the possibilities for healing in all aspects of our lives. Those of you who are familiar with Dr. Siegel's writings, lectures and seminars know that he is not only talking about physical healing, but healing of relationships, attitudes, priorities and goals in life. He uses many techniques to assist patients in their journey to wellness: dreams, drawings, imagery, visualization, meditation, positive thinking and support groups. At the end of the book he includes meditation exercises.

From Victim to Victor by Harold H. Benjamin Ph.D. He explodes the myth that an individual with cancer must accept passively whatever fate has in store. Dr. Benjamin reminds the patient that he can do a lot to maintain or restore physical well-being. While no substitute for professional treatment, the techniques of guided imagery, support groups and personal active participation in the recovery process can support and enhance good medical care. He encourages the belief and hope that one's own activities can have a beneficial effect on the recovery process and improve quality of life.

You Can Heal Your Life by Louise Hay The author tells a personal story of tragedy, abuse and cancer, and how she gradually overcame her feelings of low self-esteem and became a metaphysical counselor and a leader in a New Age group. Although I do not subscribe to her philosophy, I realize that cancer patients find healing in many different ways.

Forgive and Forget by Lewis B. Smedes. Perhaps the most difficult thing to attain in our lives is the ability to forgive ourselves for past mistakes and to forgive others who have hurt us. We need to examine our thoughts and feelings carefully to see if the inability to forgive is restricting our ability to live life with love. Read this book. It will have a profound effect on how you view yourself and others.

A Pretty Good Person: What It Takes to Live with Courage, Gratitude and Integrity OR When Pretty Good Is As Good As You Can Be by Lewis B. Smedes. This author has a special knack for going to the heart of problems that get in the way of our ability to live our lives with joy and love. Smedes believes that deep inside of every human being is the longing to be a good person. He thinks that most of us are muddling through on our road to developing what he calls character. Although we may never reach the goals we are seeking, Smedes believes we become a better person for the effort. In this book, he discusses gratitude, courage, integrity, taking charge of our lives, grace and love.

Choices: Making Right Decisions In A Complex World by Lewis B. Smedes. This is a very thought provoking book with many insightful strategies to help us lead a life that is happier and more productive. I like this author because he does not pretend to have all the answers. Instead, he examines the pros and cons of behavior as it relates to ourselves and others. In other words, he gives us some guidelines to think about and perhaps incorporate in our own lives.

Other books by Lewis B. Smedes are *How Can It Be All Right When Everything Is All Wrong?* And *Caring and Commitment.*

Healing Words by Larry Dossey M.D. Dr. Dossey was a practicing physician for many years. After he began to pray for and with his cancer patients, he found the healing effects were often astounding. Eventually, he decided to devote his life to researching the power of prayer in the practice of medicine. This book details many of the research studies that have been completed. Dossey says, "True believers think prayer is always helpful and skeptics think it is worthless. Skeptics would say if the cancer disappears it is coincidence."

The Healing Path of Prayer by Ron Roth with Peter Occhiogrosso. Ron Roth was a practicing Catholic priest for many years who discovered he had healing powers. This book is a treasure, well written and convincing. The author tells a compelling story of his experiences and guides all of us on how to pray in order to tap into the healing energy of God. If we all practiced what Roth teaches, it would lead us to serenity and a happier existence.

Disciplines of the Spirit by Howard Thurman. Dr. Thurman was a poet, mystic, philosopher and theologian. He authored more than twenty books. This one discusses commitment, growing in wisdom and stature, suffering, prayer and reconciliation. This book helped me more the second time I had cancer than any other I read, especially the chapter on suffering.

Ageless Body, Timeless Mind by Deepak Chopra. Dr. Chopra writes eloquently on the mind/body connection. He believes that society has conditioned us to believe that we are inevitable victims of sickness, aging and death. In this book, he tells us that it is possible to reverse these assumptions as the mind has the ability to influence every cell in our body. He emphasizes that we have to do our part by living a healthy lifestyle. Chopra also discusses the need for love in our life and how it lifts us up and transforms us.

Molecules of Emotion by Candace Pert Ph.D. This is a fascinating story of the author's professional and personal life. It tells of her struggles in a mostly male field of scientific research. She was the scientist who, in collaboration with her partner, proved scientifically the connection between the mind and the body. She discusses the importance of the immune system and how our emotions affect the efficiency of our physical health.

Remarkable Recovery: What Extraordinary Healings Tell Us About Getting Well and Staying Well by Caryle Hirshberg and Marc Ian Barasch. The authors of this book set out to examine why some cancer patients survive against all odds. The examples they present have often been called "miracles" or "spontaneous remissions". Hirshberg and Barasch interviewed all of these patients in an attempt to find a common thread in their survival. From what they learned in these interviews, they believe that the mind/body connection can no longer be ignored by the medical profession. This book should be an inspiration to anyone who has cancer. It gives us story after story of patients who beat the odds. It calls for a new approach to medicine; one that takes into account all aspects of the patient, physical and emotional.

The Power Within—True Stories of Exceptional Cancer Patients Who Fought Back With Hope by Wendy Williams. The stories of the ten patients in this book are not intended to tell you how to cure cancer although each goes into great detail about their treatments. They do show the wide range of possibilities in our lives. The interviews with these particular patients offer proof that anything can happen after the diagnosis of cancer and that miracles do occur. Without exception, these are examples of patients who did not deny the diagnosis but they did deny the verdict. Each story has something valuable to teach us. The people in this book are sometimes fearful, sometimes angry, sometimes filled with grief, but they are never passive.

Getting Well Again by O. Carl Simonton, M.D., Stephanie Matthew-Simonton and James L. Creighton. The authors of this book were one of the first medical persons to recognize the mind/ body connection in the treatment of cancer. A very helpful book as you learn to participate in your wellness.

The Healing Journey by O. Carl Simonton, M.D. and Reid Henson with Brenda Hampton. This book is an extension of Simonton's years of research as to how the mind can be used to influence the body most effectively. He tells us that he has learned that the power of the mind goes far beyond what he first imagined. Working with patients he discovered another dimension that influences wellness and that is spirit. Simonton believes that spirit gives persons a resource that cannot be reached through traditional psychological approaches. This book also includes letters from a patient, Reid Henson, detailing how he changed his life and survived after being diagnosed with hairy cell leukemia and told he didn't have long to live.

Anatomy of an Illness by Norman Cousins. The author's account of how he helped cure himself of a fatal disease.

Head First by Norman Cousins. Norman Cousins was a pioneer in recognizing the importance of the mind/body connection in the process of healing. This book chronicles the exciting years at UCLA as Cousins explored, with the medical staff and patients, the possibilities that we do have a great deal of control over the state of our health and well being.

Fire in the Soul, A New Psychology of Spiritual Optimism by Joan Borysenko, Ph.D. Joan Borysenko, with her background in psychology, combines her knowledge in that field with a strong belief in the spiritual side of every person. In her counseling and teaching she emphasizes the necessity of letting go of the past in order to move into the future. The author has an impressive educational background, but tells us that she has learned the most from her own personal trials and those of friends, family and clients. In other words, we learn by living. She points out that regrets and resentments are a major source of unhappiness that can keep us stuck for a lifetime. In the search for meaning, there is a discussion of good things coming out of tragedy: better understanding, more compassion, bonding of individuals to name a few of the positive things that can come out of suffering.

This is a long list and still does not begin to cover all of the informative and inspirational books available. I would urge you to pick one and get started by reading a little each day. I can guarantee you it will help.

Rules for Living with Joy

Thank God every day for being alive.

Express love every day.

Learn from your mistakes, release them and go on.

Forgive yourself and others.

Do an act of kindness without expecting anything in return.

Reach out to those in need.

Read something inspirational.

Look at the world of nature around you and enjoy.

Express gratitude for the good things in your life. It's hard to be depressed when you are counting your blessings.

Be a good listener.

Take time for yourself.

Don't sweat the small stuff.

Laugh—it's good for your health and your soul.

Do It Anyway

Written by Mother Theresa

People are often unreasonable, illogical and self-centered. Forgive them anyway.

If you are kind, people may accuse you of selfish, ulterior motives. Be kind anyway.

If you are successful, you will win some false friends and some true enemies. Succeed anyway.

If you are honest and frank, people may cheat you. Be honest and frank anyway.

What you spend years building, someone could destroy overnight. Build anyway.

If you find serenity and happiness, they may be jealous. Be happy anyway.

The good you do today, people will often forget tomorrow. Do good anyway.

Give the world the best you have, and it may never be enough. Give the world the best you have got anyway.

You see, in the final analysis, it is between you and God. It was never between you and them anyway!

Just for Today

Author Unknown

Just for today I will try to live through this day only, and not tackle my whole life problem at once. I can do something for twelve hours that would appall me if I felt that I had to keep it up for a lifetime.

Just for today I will be happy. This assumes to be true what Abraham Lincoln said, that "Most folks are as happy as they make up their minds to be."

Just for today I will adjust myself to what is, and not try to adjust everything to my own desires. I will take my "luck" as it comes, and fit myself to it.

Just for today I will try to strengthen my mind. I will study, I will learn something useful, I will not be a mental loafer, I will read something that requires effort, thought and concentration.

Just for today I will exercise my soul in three ways: I will do somebody a good turn, and not get found out; if anybody knows about it, it will not count. I will do at least two things I don't want to do—just for the exercise. I will not show anyone that my feelings are hurt; they may be hurt, but today I will not show it.

Just for today I will be agreeable. I will look as well as I can, dress becomingly, talk low, act courteously, criticize not one bit, not find fault with anything, and not try to improve or regulate anybody except myself.

Just for today I will have a program. I may not follow it exactly, but I will have it. I will save myself from two pests: hurry and indecision.

Just for today I will have a quiet half hour all by myself, and relax. During this half hour, sometime, I will try to get a better perspective of my life.

Just for today I will be unafraid. I will enjoy that which is beautiful, and will believe that as I give to the world, so the world will give to me.

Epilogue

It is a source of amazement to me that I am now 80 years old. The years have slowed me down some, but I still lead a very active life. Every day is interesting and often full of pleasant surprises. I have had to meet physical and emotional challenges over my lifetime, but there have been many good times, too. Except for the automobile accident over which I had no control and my mysterious episode with pain a year and a half ago, I have been in excellent health since 1973.

I attribute this to the wake up call I received when I was diagnosed with cancer. It made me evaluate every area of my life and make the many changes that I have described in this book.

I am a member of the generation Tom Brokaw writes about in his book *The Greatest Generation*. We didn't think of ourselves as the greatest in any way, but we were survivors.

The experience of living through the depression seems incomprehensible in today's world. There was no welfare, food stamps or government help of any kind. It was neighbor helping neighbor. At one time my father's brother who was unemployed, his wife and five children lived with us in our small house with one bathroom. To this day my sister and I cannot remember where everyone slept. I do know that there was no question of sharing what we had. We had a place to live and I don't remember ever going hungry. Life consisted of the basic necessities with no luxuries.

An education for us daughters was important to my father and somehow we managed to go to college. We lived at home and took the streetcar (since replaced by buses) across town to the University of Washington. Ben and I were married soon after graduating and left the next day for the East Coast for him to attend law school. We didn't have any money, and our families did not help with tuition or expenses. We just had a lot of faith.

We were married less than three months before Pearl Harbor and the beginning of the World War II. Ben received a commission in the Navy and was allowed to finish his first year of law school. He was in the service for five years and spent a year and a half of that time in the South Pacific on Guadacanal.

After the war, he worked eight hours a day and went to Law School nights for two straight years in order to finish. By that time, we had one child and another one born while he was in school. We lived in a small one bedroom apartment with no air conditioning in Washington, D.C. We hadn't planned it that way, but becoming a lawyer was Ben's dream and there was no question that somehow he would finish.

I never heard anyone complain about the time spent serving his country. Those fortunate enough to return, picked up the pieces of their lives, went back to school or work and tried to make up for time lost. It was a dedicated, hard working generation. Perhaps that is why we are all so grateful for what we have today.

I view my life as an interesting and challenging journey. There have been highs and lows as I imagine is true for everyone. I have been blessed with four wonderful children, their spouses and six beautiful grandchildren. I thank God every day that I have lived to see all of them grow up to be responsible adults.

References

Prescription for Living by Bernie S. Siegel, M.D.

The Healing Effect by Dale A. Matthews; Guideposts magazine, July 1999.

Prayer as Medicine by John H. Cristy; Forbes magazine, March 23, 1998.

Healing Words and the Healing Power of Prayer by Larry Dossey, M.D.; HarperCollins Publisher, Inc. 10 East 53rd Street, New York, New York 10022.

The Healing Path of Prayer by Ron Roth with Peter Occhiogrosso. Publisher, Harmony Books, a division of Crown Publishers, Inc. 201 East 53rd Street, New York, New York 10022. 1997

Disciplines of the Spirit by Howard Thurman. Published by Friends United Press, 101 Quaker Hill Drive, Richmond, IN 47374 in 1963. At the time of his death in 1981, Dr. Thurman was Dean Emeritus of Marsh Chapel, Boston University, and Chairman of the Board of Trustees of the Howard Thurman Educational Trust in San Francisco. He also served as Dean of Rankin Chapel, Howard University, Washington, D.C., as a professor at Howard University School of Religion, and as a Director of Religious Life at Morehouse and Spelman Colleges, Atlanta, Georgia. He was the founder of the first interracial interdenominational church in the United States.

Forgive and Forget by Lewis B. Smedes, professor of philosophy and integration at Fuller Graduate School of Psychology in Pasadena, California. Published by Harper & Row in 1984.

New Choices in Natural Healing edited by Bill Gottlieb and published by Prevention magazine in 1995.

Dutch Study at Vrije Univertitiet in Amsterdam by Bob Condor. Published in the Chicago Tribune.

Seniors Guide to Pain-Free Living: All-Natural DRUG FREE Relief for Everything That Hurts by Doug Dollemore and the editors of Prevention magazine. Published by Rodale in 2000.